MARK LANYON

Who Stole Grandma?

A son's memoir of love, laughter & loss

Dedicated to:

Geraldine Lanyon
Who, to me, will forever be 'Moosh'

To
Alyson Posselwhite
Moosh's daughter and my sister,
Who tried before I did
And
Geraldine Ann Kowalick
Who was named after Moosh and, with whom
Aly and I have been trying to piece together the threads of
our mothers' stories

And to
Alex, Liam, Arun, Harvey and Ayesha
Moosh's adored grandchildren

Contents

VII   Part Seven

I

Part One

HMW's Birthday Party
January 2007

1

The Call

The party was in full flow.

At that time in our life, there were always parties at our house - parties for any excuse: our birthdays, family birthdays, friends' birthdays, New Year, Diwali, you name it. I'm not keen on parties, but Her Most Wonderfulness is, so we party.

It was Her Most Wonderfulness's birthday. Not a special number, but a chance to fill the house with friends, have a drink and a catch up and let our collective hair down. The new school term had just begun. My school was in Inspection Readiness Mode, so having the distraction of a party was not such a bad thing.

As parties go, this one was going well. No one was intolerably drunk (yet), friends from our different circles were mingling sociably and people who only really ever had a chance to catch up at our parties were renewing their acquaintances.

I had not long stepped into the veranda to catch up with a group of friends from our college days and was settling into what could be hours of banter and storytelling, when HMW appeared with her worried face on.

She was waving the house phone at me, saying, "It's Alyson. She doesn't sound good."

She headed off to keep the party going.

"I can't do it Al!" were the first words I heard, followed rapidly by: "She's impossible! She just won't listen! I've put my back out trying to lift her! I can't do it!"

"Hang on a minute Aly," I stalled. "Just let me go to where we can talk properly."

Trish, Grego, TC and the others were all trying to give me as much privacy as a three by four veranda will give you, when it's crammed with fifteen people and too much furniture. Through the door to the kitchen, I could see a press of drinking bodies blocking my route to the rest of the house. That left the door to the garden.

Thankfully, space was easy to find, as there were relatively few smokers. On the downside, the reason for the absence of smokers was that it was raining and seasonally cold, it being January.

"OK, Aly, I'm here and I will be able to hear you properly. What's happened?"

From the North, the floodgates opened: "I know I wanted to do this. I know I said I could do this. But I can't. She's so unreasonable. She won't listen. She'll do what you say. You're the Golden Son! She always does what you say!"

"That's a bit harsh! She doesn't always." I muttered, very silently, to myself, while audibly I asked, "I know Moosh was a bit of a bugger about eating, but what's happened to your back?"

"It's her! She pretends that she can't move, when I know she can! She makes me pick her up and I just can't. I tried and she turned to jelly. And I couldn't hold her. And my back went! And she knows I can't, but she expects me to! And now she's in the hospital in Brotton!"

I was trying to catch my breath and it wasn't even me speaking. I was trying to catch one for Aly, too, because I intuited that the outpouring of angst was inhibiting inhalation.

"Breathe Aly," I said, as gently as possible.

"Fuck off Al!" came the anticipated invective. "It's not your back and it's not you who will be the bad daughter!"

Aly is my little sister, younger by eighteen months.
I am the first born and a boy. For reasons that neither of us have ever fully understood, but have both believed to be unfair, Aly is right: I am the Golden Son. At many points in our lives, this has made our relationship fraught, but in the months before this phone call, we had been presenting as united a front as our markedly different life circumstances would allow. United to try to manage our mother's deteriorating health needs. Since our teens, we have both called our mother, 'Moosh'.

Aly had put herself in to bat, stating that she wanted Moosh to go to live with her, 200 miles away, up in North Yorkshire. In light of recent events, both of us agreed that Moosh could not return home, because living independently at home was putting her at grave risk and had nearly killed her twice. I had argued that all of Moosh's medical support was in the Midlands, where she had lived for 20 years, since our Dad died. Aly had countered that: a) my job as a head teacher, and Ranjit's, as a language support teacher, giving children the first bricks of English to allow them to access school, prevented us from looking after Moosh at our house; that b) "they have hospitals Up North too"; and that c) there was no way that she was going to see her put into a home.

All of us, including Moosh, agreed about the 'She's not going in a home' part and I knew that Aly was right about our jobs. Aly was already a carer for Harvey, her younger, teenage son, and asserted that she was already at home 24/7 and could extend her caring role to two people, Harvey and Moosh.

Now, it seemed that it had all gone full-on belly-up, or maybe 'back-down', because of Moosh's stubbornness. I knew Aly was right. Moosh would be pushing it and demanding attention. I knew, because Moosh herself had told me some of what she got up to. She had admitted it.

"Are you there, Al?"
Aly's query brought me back to the garden. My teeth were chattering and my party shirt was soaked and clinging to me in a way that might have been attractive in my younger, fitter days, but not now that I had slipped to my more lived in, rotund form.

"Just trying to work out what to do," I assured her. "I'll come up to you. I can be there tomorrow. I'll go visit Mum and talk to her and see if I can get her to be more reasonable."

"No Al!" she butted in. "You think you can sort everything. I'm telling you that I can't do it. We need a different solution. I need to see what the social worker can do. I can't have her living here any longer. I can *not* do it!"

Shitty death! I grappled for the ability to make a useful suggestion from a brain that was slowly succumbing to hypothermia and that had, only moments before, been operating at Inane Party Banter level. I could feel our world shifting and hear walls creaking, ready to tumble.

"How soon can you arrange to see Mum's social worker?" I ventured. "I can try and get up during the week. School will let me come. How good is the social worker?"

"Thanks Al."

She sounded horribly weary, and even more heartbreakingly, disconsolately guilty, but pressed on, "Thanks. I will ring her on Monday. That's the soonest. Then I'll let you know. I'm so sorry. I thought I could do this."

Trying to keep the trembling, from the cold and from my worry, out of my voice, I said, "Don't do this to yourself. You tried when I couldn't. We will get the social worker's advice and see what we come up with. We'll work something out."

"Thanks Al. I love you." I knew she was trying to hide that she was crying.

"I love you too," I shivered.

"You're freezing! Fuck off back to your party. Give my love to Ranj. I'll call you when I know something."

As I took my chattering teeth and drenched-to-the-skin rotundness back inside to a houseful of guests, who knew nothing of my conversation with Aly, I was keenly aware that the situation was serious, that the foundations of Aly's care for Mum were shifting under stress, and that I needed to act. Being a fixer, I arrogantly believed I would be able to drive north and put things right.

What I did not know, then, was that phone call, on a party night, was the catalyst to the unfolding of a whole new, entirely unplanned for, chapter of my life.

2

HMW's Decision

The main reason that I don't relish parties is that, inside my head, I am gut-wrenchingly shy. Almost none of my friends believe this personal truth, because I have learnt to disguise my shyness with a very convincing, outward facing confidence that allows me to comfortably speak to an assembly of children, staff and parents at school, or a conference of hundreds of colleagues and strangers. Faced with a room full of people with their party heads on, however, I would rather be almost anywhere else.

The second reason, but an even more significant one, is that, if the party is at our house, my list of roles includes: tidy house to a point of presentability; hide as much of Her Most Wonderfulness's clutter/detritus as possible; disguise the fact that our daughter's bedroom doubles as a lab in which she experiments with growing mould in the various cups and plates that she has accumulated; shopping; food prep; arrange drinks counter (very extensive); move furniture; clear the veranda to create additional space; critically, turn the back room into a karaoke den; even more critically, turn the front room into HMW's dance space; make sure there is a smokers space in the garden; shop for any last minute items. (HMW's roles are: to witter for many days about what to wear; to change her mind about what to wear; to adorn herself in fairy lights; to radiate party atmosphere and drag people off to dance.) My list continues with: be complimentary about HMW's outfit; be complimentary about HMW's final choice of outfit; find batteries for HMW's fairy lights; answer the door in a welcoming manner; be the drinks facilitator (in fairness, I love this role and excel at it); first tidy up (on the night); second tidy up (the morning after); provide bacon sarnies to combat hangovers.

Surreally, having returned from my conversation with Aly, and changed from my sodden clothes into dry ones, I slipped straight into the fun of being drinks facilitator.

To HMW's queries about the phone call, I responded, "It's just Mum. We can sort it out."

I glided, seamlessly, into first tidy up. I was sorely tempted to emulate our friend, Kenny, who is my all-time Party Hero, for the wonderful reason that he has been known to signal that the party is over by unsubtly ushering guests to their coats with the hoover. HMW must have sensed that it wasn't as simple as 'just Mum', because, most unusually, she mucked in with tidying up and everything was done and dusted before we headed upstairs.

Once in bed, despite post-party weariness, HMW turned to me and said, very simply, "So tell me."

Just as in the garden in the rain, when talking to Aly, I had sensed the shift in my world, I guessed that, by sharing Aly's news, I was about to catalyse emotions and actions in my

9

wife/best friend that might alter our home, our family set up and the dynamic of our twenty-year-old marriage.

Little did I realise quite where this would take us all.

I outlined Aly's predicament, either starting or finishing with, "She's done. She can't do it any longer."

I saw Ranjit's eyes shift out of focus, as her mind disappeared inwards.

In the silence, I must have dropped off to sleep, because I was woken by Ranjit saying, "We'll have her here. She can come to live with us."

We had talked about this before, extensively, when we came to the realisation that Moosh was not safe on her own. We had discussed all of the very grown up pros and cons. We knew that part of us wanted to be supportive, but had allowed ourselves to convince one another of the maths; our jobs and our roles as parents mitigated against the additional commitment. We had tried to puzzle out the domestic algebra of catering for two different generations of our family: our eldest's music gigs, which were a big part of our lives; our middle one's football academy, twice weekly training and matches; the fact that our youngest was already not getting enough of our time; all weighed against the demands of my Mum's health. In so many ways, Aly shouldering the responsibility for Mum had solved our guilty equation for us.

I reminded Ranjit of all of this, while a flickering part of me was rejoicing.

"It's late. I'm pooped. I can't think about this properly. Let's talk tomorrow," I suggested, wanting to give her wriggle room, room that I was already hoping she would not need.

"I love you."

"Today," Ranjit whispered. "It's already tomorrow. I love you too. Night."

I'm not sure that I slept much, as part of me was a-jitter with excitement. Another part was terrified, utterly, bowel-liquefyingly terrified. I went downstairs early and pseudo-watched Match Of The Day, while pondering and mulling and arguing with myself and revisiting the equation from every angle.

The morning after a party in our house is normally, necessarily, slow, but at the first signs of life from our bedroom, I had the kettle on, the breakfast on a tray with Ranjit's cup of tea, and I was on my way upstairs, looking for signs of any lingering hangover that might prevent us from continuing our conversation. Brilliantly, there were none.

"I haven't changed my mind. We'll have her here. Geraldine can come to live with us," Ranjit declared, before I had even walked around to her side of our bed.

Half-heartedly, I opened my mouth to mount the rebuttal that I felt I should make.

Ranjit stopped me: "Mark, I'm Indian, remember. This is how Indian families work. Ever since I was a little girl, I expected to look after my husband's family. I was raised to be ready for it.

"We can do this. I will ask if I can reduce my days at school, so that I am home more often, and we can explore what help we can get through social services. The children will help, I'm sure."

And there it was: a decision that I'd spent all night hoping for, but had not wanted to press for.

11

Ranjit *is* Indian, but our choice of being a mixed-race couple went against the expectations of her family and her culture: that her husband would be chosen for her and her marriage arranged.

Our desire to have a love marriage and to build our little mixed-race family has resulted in us having little to do with the wider Indian community. In knowingly breaking the rules, we hoped that we could reshape her family's expectation and, over time, gain the acceptance that we were seeing in some Sikh families. Years down the line, this had not happened and so we have lain in the bed we've made, separated from Ranjit's culture, for fear of giving further offence or adding greater hurt.

Despite all of this, at her core, Ranjit's values are deeply embedded. Her sense of duty to her elders has never been lost. At many points in the past, she had stated that one day Moosh should come to live with us.

"How can we live on less money?" I asked, determined to test her.

"We're comfortable. Look at us. We're good," she reassured me.

"Worse comes to worst, we'll live on dahl!" she added with a chuckle.

This has always been our line, when we make a financial decision: house buying = dahl; car buying = dahl; starting a family = dahl. A diet of dahl is the solution to all financial worries.

"God, I love you!" I declared, beginning to naively grasp that our lives were set on a new course.

"So you should!" she beamed.

If she had any sense, that morning, of the unfolding of the

years ahead, she hid it.

Over more tea and snuggled up against the cold, we talked pragmatically through needs and hurdles and options: what did we think Moosh needed; what was she able to do for herself; where would she sleep; what might she like in her room; what would we need to bring from her house; what did we need to heed from Aly's experience; what did I need to ask the social worker.

On and on we talked, into the early afternoon, problem solving together.

At some point, around the seventh cup of tea, I sat up abruptly, turned to Ranjit and asked, "What if she doesn't want to come?"

3

Road Trip To Brotton

And so it was that, on the following Wednesday, I left school at lunchtime to resume my now familiar battle with the M1, praying that the stretch past Meadowhall would somehow discern the urgency of my trip and not be too tediously stand still. As it turned out, I only needed one stop to pick up a hot chocolate, and Sheffield was kind to me for only the second time in my life, so I was on the A174 skirting past the southern reaches of Middlesbrough in very good time, looking out for my usual landmarks.

Until that day, I had never even noticed Brotton on my trips to Aly and Neil's in Loftus.

I had no idea that it was the birthplace of the designer of *The Spirit Of Ecstasy*, the Rolls Royce emblem; or that its ironstone mine, Lumpsey, was so significant in World War One that it had warranted military defence; or that its history predated the Domesday Book, back to the Roman signalling station that has long since fallen in to the sea.

Brotton was always lost through my fixation on spotting

the big mining sheave wheel on the Kilton roundabout, which would announce that I only had 2.5 miles left of my near-200 mile trip. Never once had I looked north towards the village.

Now, heading to see Moosh, that sheave wheel told me not to head onwards, but to turn left, and there it was: Brotton, or at least Upper Brotton.

Having made such good time, I drove straight past the hospital, putting off the moment, using the valid excuse of finding something to eat. Although my stomach was in coiling knots and I had no appetite, I forced myself to eat, telling myself that my body needed fuel to keep me going through whatever the afternoon held.

I made my jitters worse by taking out the list that I had prepared: questions for the hospital; for the social worker; for Aly; and questions for Moosh. I read them through. It was a sensible list. All of the questions would give answers to help us to understand the situation. It was only the last question on the list that had burnt a hole in my pocket for 196 miles: it was the one that I could not guess the answer to.

Being used to the size of the city of Birmingham and the borough of Sandwell, my sandwich hunting tour of the upper and lower parts of Brotton left me stunned that a village of its size would have its own hospital, but it did, and I could no longer put off entering it. Not only does it have one, but, despite its much smaller scale, the hospital radiated efficiency and welcome. I was quickly taken through to see Moosh and assured that she was doing well.

By this point in her life, I should have been used to seeing her in a hospital bed, but seeing her surrounded by unhomely paraphernalia, she may have looked more forlorn than I had seen her since our father passed away, twenty years earlier.

"I've spoilt it all, haven't I? Alyson doesn't want me."

No passing Go and collecting £200, no gentle build up, she just took us straight into the painful conversation.

"Ma, it's not like that. Things have got difficult. Alyson's back is giving her a huge amount of pain. No one is saying that it is your fault, but her back can not cope with everything that you need her to do for you."

I attempted an initial tack away from the fractured mother-daughter relationship, by focussing on the physical.

"Her back has never been the strongest. She and I talked about whether it would be up to this, before you came up here, but she thought that she would be able to cope. I don't think she realised how much physical strength she would need and how much she would need to help you to get about."

"And now she doesn't want me," Moosh insisted.

"It's not that she doesn't want you, but it's not just her back. She is feeling very hurt too. You haven't been entirely fair," I could see her beginning to bridle as I tacked back to the emotional damage that had been done. "You have been very demanding, not always fairly. You have made her do things for you that you didn't need. You have pretended that you couldn't do things that you really could. What you told the social worker has really upset her."

I did not tell her about Alyson's fury when Moosh had demonstrated to the social worker that she could stand, sit and mobilise, precisely the things that she was demanding assistance with. Nor did I tell her that Alyson had excused herself from the room at the point that Moosh answered the social worker's question about feeding by stating that she was perfectly able to feed herself, but liked to make her daughter do it.

I certainly omitted the fact that Alyson's comment to the social worker was, "I'm going out for a cigarette, because, if I punch my mother in front of a social worker, it's not going to look very good, is it?"

The fact was that the fury and hurt were there. Alyson was deeply affronted that, in the lead up to the social worker's visit, Moosh had been falling over and banging into walls, apparently unable to move without assistance and needing to be lifted back up, supported bodily, or even carried, but in front of the social worker she had transformed into a performing seal, touching her toes and bouncing round like an eighteen-year-old at a rave.

The empathetic hug that the social worker had given Aly, when she found her in the kitchen, broken, had been much needed and greatly appreciated, but could not remove the hurt or bridge the gap. Nor could the social worker's assurances that she regularly saw such behaviour in elderly clients, who, feeling under threat of perceived incarceration, suddenly, and temporarily, regain previously long-lost faculties.

I did not tell her that Aly's pained summary to me, after the social worker's visit was, "Al, she is highly demanding and utterly contrary. She is refusing to cooperate, and she is refusing outside care. She wants only me, Neil or Liam. What she really wants is for me to do everything for her. She enjoys it. She won't let me get any help with caring for her and so there is no respite. Harv needs me too!"

Instead of telling her any of that, I asked, "What do you want to happen, Ma?"

Her answer floored me: "I want to be loved."

"That's horrible, Ma! Alyson has done nothing but love you! And Neil and Liam have, too! She has created a lovely space for you, a space full of love! She brought you here, knowing that Harvey needs her too and knowing that I thought it would be too much for her and for them. I'm sorry to say that, from what I can see, you have been much more demanding than you needed to be, probably because you have absolutely loved having all the attention, but you have pushed it way too far."

"What should I do?" she asked, looking at me intently. "What do you think I should do?"

Looking at her face, I could see that my words had struck home. She looked riven with guilt, but I knew that she had burnt her bridges, irreparably. There was no way back for her at Alyson's.

It was time for the question on the bottom of my list, but first I suggested, "It might help to apologise."

At that moment, I was far from certain that an apology would be welcome, but I needed Moosh to be ready for the moment, should it come.

I thought I saw the flicker of a protest come to her lips, but by the time the words emerged they carried contrition and awareness, "I will. If she'll allow me."

I reached across and held her hand, and asked my question, "Ma, will you come to live with us? We'd like you to."

Again, she stared at me, before crumpling, "But it's Ranjit's house."

"It's our house, Ma," I answered, "but it was Ranjit who suggested it. What do you think?"

She attempted levity, "I'd better behave hadn't I?"

18

"Is that a yes?" I asked.

Her 'Yes, please,' was a mixture of surprised gratitude and a crestfallen *mea culpa*.

I was delighted that she wanted to come to live with us, but I did nothing to remove her remorse, as I hoped that it would help to modify her interactions with Aly over the coming weeks, and be a stimulus to her recognising the efforts that Aly had made, and prompt her into at least trying to rebuild those incinerated bridges.

My list of questions included only the two for Moosh: 1) What did she want? and 2) Would she come to live with us?

All the other questions were for the hospital, to clarify her condition and her ongoing medical needs; for the social worker, to gain advice as to how to care for her; and for Alyson, to find out whether she would have Moosh back for a finite period of time.

From the hospital I learned that there had been no major deterioration in Moosh's Parkinson's Disease. She was somewhat frailer, but there was nothing to prevent her from being discharged.

The social worker was just as fabulous and supportive as Aly had described. She identified the level of care that Moosh would be able to access, should she stay at Aly's, which in the first instance included an allocation of carer's support to alleviate the burden that Aly was shouldering. She was clear that Moosh's files would be efficiently forwarded to parallel services in Sandwell and identified equipment that might benefit Moosh, moving forward. She also volunteered to provide me directly with any further information I required in meeting with her Sandwell counterparts, and liaising with them in the weeks and months ahead.

Crucially, Aly was amenable. She was still hurt, deeply affronted and tautly angry, but she was willing to accept the provision of a carer and the establishment of a timetabled routine to afford me the time to make arrangements at home.

I drove back towards the M1 via the hospital to let Moosh know what had been agreed.

All she wanted to know was, "Will Alyson forgive me?"

"You will have to try to make sure that she does," I advised. "It would help us all, massively, if you think about helping the people, who are trying to help you. Believe me, when you come to us, the only way it will work is if you work with us."

Driving home, I had no idea whether she would listen, or whether she and Alyson would be able to navigate their way back to one another, but I had to hope.

II

Part Two

Shakespeare Road
Before October 2006

4

No 1 Childminder

On the night of my rain-soaked conversation with Aly, Moosh was just short of her 79th birthday.

As Her Most Wonderfulness and I embraced the notion of Moosh coming to live with us, and made preparations, part of us puzzled, painfully, over whether there were signs that we had been blind to.

We spent many weekend mornings, over breakfast in bed (almost the only time in the week when we could snatch time to talk), dissecting the past in search of clues that we had missed, or opportunities we might have taken, that could have prevented us from reaching this point.

We found precious few.

Moosh had remained vital and active well into her 70s, a ball of energy capable of galivanting across the globe.

Having lost our father in her late fifties, she embraced travel, heading first to Turkey with Elisabeth, a dear friend from her expat life in Iran, and then to Canada to stay with Evelyn and Jim, also friends from her years in Iran, where she took part in the Sun Run in her sixties. Her faith saw her join pilgrimages to Rome and the Holy Land. Then, most stunning and joyful of all, her reconnection with her sister, Marguerite, after an interval of 47 years, triggered her last and longest international jaunt, to stay with her in Adelaide for a fortnight - Moosh was 74.

We have just followed in her footsteps to Australia, in our mid-50s, and come home utterly knackered, but looking back to her visit, we had not worried about her going, so must have judged her health to be up to the Antipodean adventure, or maybe not even felt, yet, that it was our position to judge - there appeared to be no need to.

Similarly, in her 70s, she was still loving the pottery classes that she had joined not long after moving to Smethwick. Despite her capacity for incredible insularity, she would head off each week, confidently taking the bus to West Bromwich, where she thrilled at fashioning all manner of pots, decorating and glazing them and loving the act of bestowing them as gifts.

Recently, I was rearranging some ornaments on a bookcase at home and was slightly stunned (and tearfully overjoyed) to see her initials neatly etched into the base of a pot that I have admired for years. I had entirely forgotten that it was one of hers, thinking that we had bought it.

Some of her pottery was really rather good, but far more importantly, she loved being part of those classes. She had first joined them after Dad died and they gave her a way back into the world, something to look forward to in the week, a reason to get up on a Wednesday, a way of connecting with people, however transiently, and a way of rediscovering her zest for life.

The first indication from Moosh that she might be suffering some age-related decline was her admission that she was having difficulty with some of the manipulation tasks at pottery class.

Early on, when I had admired a thrown pot, she was open about the fact that it had been thrown by her teacher with her adding the decorative flourishes. It was not lack of skill *per se*, that prevented her from throwing her own pots on a wheel, but more a lack of dexterity caused by arthritis, the effects of which she revealed she had been struggling with for several years. She was very *'c'est la vie'* as she told me that she had been having cortisone injections to reduce the pain and allow her a greater degree of flexibility. She hinted at arthritic pain in her hips, but was far more concerned about having her pot throwing curtailed, being restricted to slab and coil pots. Such was her level of fierce independence that she had attended appointments and sought treatment without ever feeling any need to divulge her difficulties to us.

Her matter of fact approach to her arthritis and her determination that she could live her independent life reassured me, but I began to look more closely at her, as she went about her daily tasks, pottering in her garden, making drinks in her kitchen, popping to the shop around the corner for biscuits. She was, admittedly, more than a little slower than the woman I used to have races with, but amply able to nip around.

Crucial to her, she was not only able to function in her own home, but was able to be the Number One Childminder. She relished this role. It was also valuable, even critical, to us. On the one hand, it freed Her Most Wonderfulness to return to school and, at Moosh's insistence, was entirely *gratis*. On the other, and of much greater significance to us, we recognised, very early, the wonderful impact that she had on her grandchildren.

She had been in her 60s, when her first grandson, Alex, became the centre of her universe, joined less than two months later by Liam. Aly's house and ours were the second and third corners of an equilateral triangle stretching a mile from her house, a proximity intentionally created by our father, who bought her house in Shakespeare Road knowing that he was mortally ill. Several times every week, Moosh would visit each of our homes to lavish affection on her two grandsons.

When Alex was one and Ranjit finally admitted that she might have to go back to her job at school, Moosh stepped (leapt) in for two and a half days every week during term time. Alex benefitted in ways that we never imagined possible, far beyond simple care. Moosh would walk everywhere with him, first pushing his buggy, then with him toddling along holding her hand, and finally with him in full control of his legs, but still holding hands adoringly. They talked incessantly, first she to him and then together, but never, ever, baby talk. From his earliest days, she began imparting knowledge, with him a thirsty, unquenchable sponge.

On their walks she pointed out and named every different tree in gardens and parks. He quickly learned to recognise tree shape and leaf shape, both close up and from a distance. It became one of his first party pieces, dazzling adults with knowledge that most of them lacked. More conventionally, she taught him about dinosaurs and he was voracious, learning to recognise dinosaurs of land, sea and air that I had never known, devouring books in the process, identifying them from their claws and teeth, she beaming proudly all the while. She stunned me, utterly, when he showed that he could also identify pretty much any car with just a glimpse of a distinguishing feature, such as a headlight: she had learned all of their names so that she could feed his fascination and he could expand his car knowledge to encyclopaedic proportions.

She believed that he could do anything, which was how she came to bestow the gift that he has carried through his life. At the first indication of a musical ability, she took him under her encouraging wing, guiding him and gently stretching him – he was playing Mozart proficiently before he turned three, taught entirely by her.

When Arun erupted into the world, we judged that, with his boundless accident-prone energy, looking after the two of them, just two and a half years apart in age, might be too exhausting for Moosh. This time, when Ranjit was arranging childcare in the lead up to her return to school, she asked her friend, Claire, to be Arun's childminder. The arrangement worked perfectly in almost every respect, with Claire quickly being dubbed *Scary Clairy*, in Arun's mischievous way. The only drawback being that Arun never had the same opportunity to spend those early life hours and hours with his grandmother.

By the time Ayesha was one, and Ranjit was once again deciding that she should return to the classroom, Arun was in Reception at school and well settled with Scary Clairy. Moosh once again took on the role of sharing the week with Ranjit, reverting to her two and a half days a week of childcare, but now pushing Ayesha in the buggy as she walked Alex to and from school, and then looking after the pair of them until Ranjit returned home with Arun. It worked well and we were enormously grateful.

Our construct of Arun only joining his brother and sister after his stays with Scary Clairy meant that Moosh rarely had all three children in her care, but, in those moments, a loving anarchy took over, one in which her role as arbiter of good behaviour disintegrated into joyous Grandma-led subversion of mine and Ranjit's rules. The best example of which was The Radiator Incident.

In our first year in our new house, there was a period of a couple of weeks when we began to notice a disturbing odour of rankness in the kitchen. We emptied the bin, without improvement. We checked the kitchen for forgotten tubs of leftovers, but found nothing. We spent time with our noses in every cupboard, but still found nothing.

Over the next few days, we deduced that the pong was worse when the heating was on. The kitchen radiator was four feet long and powerful, belting out luxurious heat. Eventually, one teatime, I found myself crawling on my hands and knees following the smell to the very hot, very pungent radiator. When I peered behind, I was treated to the nauseating sight of mouldering pizza, sandwiches and Lord only knows what else, stuffed down the back of the radiator; it was not a small amount – it was months' worth, brimming to almost its very top (two and a half feet), all along its full four foot length.

Entirely unjustly, I targeted Arun, as Ayesha was still a toddler and Alex was out of the room, and began to interrogate him.

Hearing my angry enquiry about why he'd been putting his

food behind the radiator and my beginning of the lecture about starving children that she had used on me as a child, Moosh blithely interjected, "Don't blame Arun, poor child: it's my fault."

As my jaw gaped and Arun grinned his innocence, Moosh offered the following rationale: "When the children can't finish their food, I know that you will insist that they eat everything on their plates, just like your Dad used to make you (she omitted that she also used to). When Ranjit sees their food in the bin, she gets cross. So, we make sure it's out of sight."

She was unmoved by my flabbergasted exclamation of, "Out of sight? But it's festering and it stinks!"

Instead, she calmly twinkled, "But at least the children have not been unhappy."

And, in so doing, secured her legend status in the eyes of all three of our children.

By now, Moosh's No 1 Childminder role had become considerably elongated as she was frequently travelling to Leighton Buzzard, jumping on and off buses and trains, so that she could help with looking after Harvey and spend time with Liam.

Oddly, she kept her involvement with Aly's family and my family very separate. In all of the nineteen years from our father's death to her stay in Loftus there was not one single occasion on which she invited us all to her house, despite us all living just one mile from one another. So, very often, we would have no clue that Moosh was or had been on one of her childminding missions, unless it slipped out inconsequentially in conversation. She was, in many ways, a free spirit who simply made herself available for her five grandchildren in the diversely individual ways that they needed her.

Arun continued to go to childminders until he joined Alex at secondary school. While Alex continued to be the startlingly polite product of Moosh's tutelage throughout school, Arun turned feral and, much like a very independent tom cat, would find his way home when he needed feeding. Although they both still basked in her affection, neither of them had any need of the house-based childcare that Moosh had given them in their younger years, which allowed her to lavish time on Ayesha.

Moosh always professed to being far more comfortable with boys, nevertheless she doted on Ayesha and proudly took her to and from school into her junior school years, keeping up the habit of continual chat that had so benefitted Alex. She had now been a fixture on the Barclay Road school run for nine years and, despite her reserve, was on nodding and greeting terms with many of the home owners that she and Ayesha passed on route and many of the parents, mainly mothers, who were on the same run.

It was one of the mothers who approached Ranjit on one of her pickup days to ask, "Is Ayesha's grandma OK?"

Immediately concerned, Ranjit replied that we thought she was, to which the mother explained, "It is just that we noticed that she seems to be walking more slowly, heavily, as if she is finding it harder. We know that she is a very proud lady, so did not want to intrude by asking her, but I thought that I would mention it to you."

Ranjit, who prides herself on being vigilant about the needs of her family, Moosh included, reproved herself for having missed such a detail, but, in sharing the conversation with me, asked whether I had noticed Moosh finding walking difficult, adding that, very occasionally, she thought Moosh was shuffling. I hadn't, so we both blamed ourselves for not taking time to be more attentive.

I asked Moosh, who was indignant, feeling that people were talking about her behind her back and questioning her capacity to fulfil a role that she loved. She was immediately deeply concerned, extrapolating from our worries, that she may not be allowed to continue to be No. 1 Childminder. She shared that, yes, her hips were often uncomfortable and that her doctor had diagnosed bursitis, an inflammation of the fluid filled sacs that cushion the joints. She was, however, quietly adamant that although slower, she could still take Ayesha to and from school.

Whether fully assured or taking the easy option, we were happy for Moosh to continue, and grateful that she wanted to.

Months later, it was Ayesha who told us that Moosh had fallen on the way to school and had to be helped up by other school runners. She asked what was wrong with Grandma.

Talking to our daughter, still only 8, it became clear that she was aware that something was not quite right and, moreover, had been for some time. I was certain that she was unintentionally complicit with Moosh in hiding this. Realising that she was very maturely troubled about Moosh's wellbeing, but also disconcerted by being made to break her grandmother's confidence, I tried not to press.

However, it was clear that, without us having noticed, a key facet of their roles had reversed: something had stolen her beloved Grandma, the woman who had been such a major part of her early years. Ayesha had, of her own volition, adopted the caring, protective role and, out of love, first held her silence and now expressed her concern.

The conversation with Moosh was brutal.

I was neither unkind nor harsh in explaining to her that we felt that it was safer for her and for Ayesha that we find someone else to act as childminder. The brutality was in the impact: Moosh was bereft, with a role that she relished removed, her sense of purpose withdrawn.

We promised that she would be coming around every week and that we would still rely on her for babysitting, we only wanted to reduce the risk caused by her walking quarter of a mile to school and quarter of a mile back, twice a day, removing three thousand steps, any one of which might lead to a stumble and a fall. We explained that we did not want her to be injured or for Ayesha to find herself in a position where she felt that she had to try lift her. Not one thing we said altered the fact that Moosh felt diminished.

Her hurt feelings notwithstanding, we were true to our word: we did include Moosh in every one of our family events and she frequently came around for dinner. She did babysit regularly, in the safer confines of our home.

Things were never broken between us; she never reproached us and she forgave us almost instantly, but both she and Ayesha lost all those hours of mornings and afternoons of the togetherness and love they had shared on their walks to and from school.

5

The Last Train

The moment at which we switch from being protected by our parents to being their protector is different in every family and in each child-parent relationship. For some, the moment never comes. For example, I never became our Dad's protector, he died too soon. However, the very moment he passed away, I became Moosh's.

Ranjit and I had been for a much needed half-term minibreak, admiring the Roman and Georgian beauty of Bath. We were newlyweds, in our first year of marriage, but needing a freshener after the, always long, first half-term of the year. Answering an insistent early morning knock on the door of our B&B room, I found our best man, Steve, ashen.

To my repeated demands as to what brought him from Bristol to Bath before breakfast time, he would only say, "I need you to ring Alyson."

In a mixture of frustration and mounting fear, I went in search of the gentleman host of the B&B. My worry was heightened by the kid gloves with which he received my request to use the phone. He showed me into his private office space, just off the Reception, and seated me, before leaving me to my privacy, with a clear look of pity.

The "Al?" with which Aly answered my call was a wet sob.

Despite her tears, she did a typically Aly job of communicating the facts. Dad had phoned Moosh to say that he was experiencing terrible abdominal pains and that he had rung the ambulance. On their arrival, finding their knocks unanswered, the paramedics had summoned the police to gain entry to the house. They found Dad, collapsed in the living room, beyond help, his last cigarette having burned a ciggie-long hole in one of Moosh's beloved Chinese rugs.

Guilt rushed in. Moosh was at ours, babysitting the kittens that Dad had recently bought for us. He had known that he was ill, and the kittens, Aisha and Chiké, were his furry grandchild surrogates. I swear his eyes twinkled lovingly for the few months that he knew them, and that the number of times that he and Moosh travelled by train from Shrewsbury to Birmingham increased so that he could visit them not us. His last visit to them was when he accompanied Moosh on her trip down for two days of kitten-sitting, to allow us our mini-break, before he headed home, alone, to meet a friend for his swansong bender. Because of his grandkittens, Moosh was not with him when he died.

Far exceeding his best man duties, Steve drove us first to his parents in Bristol, then to collect a Bristolian college friend. Steve had driven us all down, earlier in the week and now, sombrely, he returned us to Smethwick, to Moosh and to my new role.

From the second we walked through our front door, a key

dynamic shifted and my new position was clear.

In Moosh's way of looking at the world, I was now head of the household, simply by virtue of gender. It mattered not a jot to her that it was not a role that I held the requisite skills or experience for. She looked to me for guidance on procedural household matters that I did not deal with in my and Ranjit's home; things that, in our set up, Ranjit always took the lead on and I had no interest in. Similarly she sought assurance on decisions that had not even been Dad's, they had always been hers alone.

In truth, over the next fortnight, it would be Ranjit and Aly, not I, who dealt with all of the onerous practicalities of funeral arrangements, navigating legalities and, crucially, continuing with the purchase of the house on Shakespeare Road that Dad was in the process of buying for Moosh.

But still, for Moosh, it was my Golden Son pedestal that was raised many notches; in her eyes, I was now her protector, a role conferred not solely, stereotypically, due to my maleness, but because I had become her consoler-in-chief, her emotional crutch. I have always been a good shoulder to cry on. It is how Her Most Wonderfulness and I became friends, me listening to her pouring out her anxieties about the expectation that she would have an arranged marriage. At my all boys boarding school, I had found a niche, maybe not as a shoulder to cry on, but as a good ear, receptive to the emotional offloading of fellow pupils, growing up away from home. And so it was with Moosh: I was there, I listened, I comforted, I filled her void – leaving the practical stuff to everyone else.

Tellingly, following Dad's passing, Moosh never comforted me once - that task fell to Ranjit. And through that single facet of our relationship, her drawing emotional strength from me rather than I from her, our future course was set, although the culmination, triggered by Moosh's deteriorating health, was still many years ahead.

Moosh did bounce back, throwing her energies into moving to her new house, rallying her confidence sufficiently to handle all of the arrangements with Pickfords herself.

She had always been the home builder and she built a new home, just for her, in the house that she would treasure as Dad's parting gift to her. It was never my home, nor Aly's, I never once slept there, nor even sat to eat at the antique dining table that had come from my paternal grandparents' house.

She independently developed new routines for herself, shopping, pottering, potterying and going to Mass. First, she tried St. Gregory's in Bearwood, but decided that it was not for her. Next, she attended St. Mary's in Harborne, where a memorial Mass had been held for Dad, but, again, felt that something was missing. Finally, she settled on the Oratory with its immense baroque grandeur, reassuring clouds of incense and the Mass in Latin.

My protective role over the next eighteen months was to be Moosh's Sunday Afternoons. She would come to us from the Oratory and we would prepare a Sunday roast. Much to the relief of our neighbour, Angela, on Sunday afternoons Moosh would project-manage the reclamation of our tiny strip of garden from the thigh-high grass and weeds that we had allowed to engulf it. Once the jungle had been tamed, she advised on the creation of small beds and their planting. Much of the rest of the week was spent doing much the same, but on a grander scale, at her considerably longer and much wider garden, all single-handedly.

Until the coming of grandchildren embedded her into our lives as Childminder Number 1, touching base on Sunday afternoons was sufficient emotional support for Moosh. She did not expect a great deal from me as her protector and demanded even less; the routine was sufficient. She continued to be independent and feisty and wandered far and wide. Once Alex was born, Moosh became tightly woven into the fabric of our home, childminding on her three days a week, babysitting frequently, but still joining us on Sundays.

Possibly, she was so close that we did not pick up the signs, nor recognise their significance.

Our decision about childminding and the school run and our emerging realisation that things were changing for Moosh still did not clip her flight feathers; she continued to leap on trains to visit Aly, although, now, this involved travelling up to Loftus, changing at Doncaster.

And so it was that one Sunday, I found myself at Birmingham New Street Station.

Contrary to deeply engrained habit, Moosh had actually told me that she would be travelling up to Loftus and asked if I wouldn't mind collecting her from the station.

Keeping my promise, I arrived in plenty of time and positioned myself facing the giant display board, showing departures and arrivals. With my back to the escalators, I ensured that I could see all of the barriers through which travellers could emerge and, as the allotted time approached, I cast my focus back and forth for a small, Paddington-like human in a duffle coat. As the minutes ticked by, I scanned and scanned in vain. Arrival time having passed, I took to looking towards the exit doors and then went out to the taxi rank: nothing. Eventually, I went down to Platform 4: nothing.

Retracing my steps, standing once again in front of the display board, I rang Aly on my new-fangled Nokia.

"She should be with you, Al," she confirmed. "Neil put her on the train on time. She had to change in Doncaster or Darlington, I'm not sure which, but she knew. I suppose that it is possible that she missed the connection."

Looking up at the board, I calculated which imminent trains might be carrying her. With all my searching around the station, it was only another thirty-five minutes until the next possibility arrived, an hour after the one on which I had been expecting her. Mildly peeved, but placated by the missed-connection rationale, I told Aly my new ETA for Moosh and that I was going in search of a Mars Bar to chomp on, and agreed to call her when Moosh eventually put in an appearance.

When Moosh did not emerge through the barrier a second time, I began to be truly anxious. I scoured the station, checking the platforms, the escalators, the taxi rank and the bus stop that would take her to Oldbury: nothing – no unclaimed little old lady. Not wanting to add to Aly's worry and preferring to avoid the conversation, I instead took the surprisingly grown up step of going in search of the station manager and asked him what the procedure would be for locating a lost human, adding that I was concerned that she had a heart condition and had, of late, been a little wobbly.

In one of those episodes of beyond-the-call-of-duty kindness that would nowadays have resulted in thousands of likes and shares on Facebook and glowing social media coverage, the station manager not only put out repeated 'lost child' calls for a missing septuagenarian, but, without first telling me, he contacted the guard on the train that had travelled from Doncaster. He also contacted the guard on the next train heading towards New Street. Replicating my search of New Street Station, the guards scoured their respective trains, from front to back and double-checked bathrooms.

He looked crestfallen when he reported to me that none of the searches had found Moosh and asked whether there was anywhere else my mother might have travelled to, or any other route that she might have taken. I undertook to call Aly, while he assured me that he would repeat the tannoy calls for Geraldine Lanyon every half hour.

Although he had told me that she had not been located on the third train to arrive, I robotically repeated my previous search pattern, to a backdrop of the promised calls. The station manager, who was running an entire station, took time to come back to find me; still nothing.

"Where the fuck can she have gone?" was Aly's stunned response to the news.

"Not to Birmingham, is my guess, Aly!" was my initial, less than helpful, rather annoyed reply.

"Sorry Al, I'm worried too," she placated. "I'm just . . ."

"I don't know where else to look!" I interrupted, trying to formulate a plan. "If she doesn't arrive soon, I am going to phone the police. Could you do the same up there? I will go back to the station manager and ask what the protocol is for a passenger who never arrives. There must be one. I'll give it one more train from up there and then call the police."

As an afterthought, I added, "If she does arrive, I'll kill her and then let you know."

Thirty minutes later, three hours after her expected arrival, the station manager emerged through the ticket barriers, immediately searching me out where I was waiting a few metres ahead of the escalators, a long, long way beyond anxious. In one hand he carried a familiar looking valise, on his face was a broad smile and his other hand guided the elbow of Moosh, who looked eminently pleased with life.

"Geraldine caught the train to Edinburgh," he explained. "Very wisely, she asked for advice, when she realised her mistake, and the guard made sure that she was put on the correct return train. Sadly, I was talking to the guards on the wrong trains, the ones already heading south. But Geraldine is here now, I'm very pleased to say."

Once I had thanked him repeatedly and Moosh had beamed at him incessantly with her coquettish 'What a nice man young man!' face on, we took our leave.

Thankfully, the time spent with him had allayed my initial impulse to throttle her, but when she was safely belted in the car, which I suddenly realised I had to help her with, I asked, "Come on, Ma, tell me what happened."

"I went to the wrong platform," she admitted, contrite. "I thought it said Birmingham on the front of the train, but it must have said, Edinburgh. They look the same, don't they?"

I hadn't turned the ignition, so was able to turn my body, directing my full, astonished, quizzical stare at her.

"They do!" she insisted, before continuing, "I got very confused. I know it. I can tell how worried you are. I'm sorry. But I did ask for help, which is good, isn't it? He was a very nice man at the station, wasn't he?"

That was the last time that Moosh travelled independently, her confidence was shot through. I hate to admit it, but I was guiltily grateful that her loss of confidence removed the need for me to ever tell her that, as her protector, I was restricting her jaunts.

6

The First Fall

Too often, in my relationship with Moosh, phone calls brought bad news. And that was the case when the phone rang at home, early one Saturday, a year or so after Moosh's last train ride.

An unfamiliar female voice asked, "Hello, is that Alistair?"

Immediately, the use of 'Alistair', rang alarm bells. This could only be to do with my mother or my sister. I am only called Alistair in their circles of friends and acquaintances.

With some trepidation, I answered, "Yes. Who is this?"

"It's Amanda. I live next door to Geraldine. Geraldine is your Mum, isn't she?"

"Hi Amanda, is there a problem? Is Mum OK?"

With gentle calmness, Amanda explained, "I think that she will be OK now, but she has been taken to hospital. I found her in her kitchen, lying on the floor under some newspaper. I had seen the light on, very late, and thought it was unusual. My Dad has a key for your Mum's house and so I was able to get in.

"We called the ambulance and they were fantastic, but they decided to take her to Dudley Road Hospital. They mentioned hypothermia. They think that they got to her in time, but that if she'd been cold for much longer, she could have died."

"Why was she in the kitchen? Has she had a fall?" I asked.

Our decision about the school run and then Moosh's train adventure had led to us researching Moosh's symptoms and to me joining Moosh at hospital appointments, both to support her and to make sure that she did not bare-faced lie to the consultants about how her illness was affecting her and the insidious deterioration she was experiencing. I lived in fear of Moosh's Parkinson's causing her to lose control and tumble. Two separate friends had already lost aged parents to complications resulting from falls.

"Alistair, I don't think she fell. It didn't look as if she had injuries caused by a fall and I don't think that the paramedics thought that was the case. It looked like she had gone to sleep under the newspaper, as if she'd used the pages as covers," shared Amanda. "I'm not being rude, but she was very dirty too."

"She'd soiled herself?" I asked.

I dreaded finding Moosh covered in excrement. I wasn't sure how I would respond in that situation, and, now, dreaded worse, that she had suffered the indignity of Amanda having found her like that.

"No. No. Not that. She was covered in soil, compost - you know, from a plant. There was an over-turned plant pot in the kitchen near her," Amanda tried to create a picture for me and then continued, "the ambulance crew said that you could go straight to the hospital. She will be in A&E still, but do you think it would be an idea to come here and collect some of your Mum's things, fresh clothes, toiletries, that sort of thing?"

I was immediately grateful that Amanda was doing the necessary thinking for me and staying so unruffled. I was only a couple of clicks away from gibbering, hoping that the calm I relied on at work would kick in soon. I was trying to visualise her face. I could see her Dad's, but only had the most fleeting recollection of meeting her a year previously. Dark hair. Pretty. Smart. Then I hit a dead end.

"Thank you so much, Amanda. I will do that. Can I pop round, when I get there? Will you be in?"

"Of course. We'll be here."

Moosh was a determinedly insular soul. When she lived in Shrewsbury, she knew the neighbours to either side, the lady over the road, who cut hair, and a few people from Church. When my father was alive, her group of acquaintances was a little wider, through him, but her deeply embedded reserve kept her circle small. Similarly, when she moved to the house that Dad had been buying for her in Smethwick, but had not lived long enough to move to with her, she formed speaking relationships with exactly the same pattern of people, either side, opposite and Church. She came across as a little up herself, being the only person on the road who referred to others by their title of Mr. or Mrs., rather than their forename.

In that context, I was enormously grateful that her neighbours were supportive and vigilant and had spotted the indicator of a light left on unusually late. From Amanda's account, it had been a close-run thing, possibly hours.

Thankful that it was the weekend, I filled Ranjit in and left her to catch up with me at the hospital, once I knew more about what would happen next. By the time I left the house for the short drive to Moosh's, I was thinking clearly.

I knocked next door and was met by Amanda, who accompanied me to Moosh's to explain further what she had found. The hallway and lounge dining room looked fine, neat and tidy, Moosh-like, leaving me entirely unprepared for the state of the kitchen. Aside from having a penchant for keeping food items eons past their use by date, Moosh was scrupulously ordered in her kitchen, as in the rest of her house, but I walked into a kitchen covered in soil. A half empty pot sat in one corner with its trailing plant very much askew. There was also soil on the sink and all across the work surface and what looked like the sheets of a whole newspaper scattered on the floor.

"That's what she was under," explained Amanda, indicating the newspaper. "It looked like she was sleeping, but her breath was very shallow and she was terribly cold. I'm not sure, but it looked like she's made a sort of bed and put herself there, under these. I don't really know. I'm just glad that Dad encouraged me to come round and check."

"So am I! Thank you so much!"

I'm certain that I thanked Amanda over and over again, before I let her out with assurances that I would let them know how Moosh was. Then, feeding off my memories of maternity trips to hospital and my own stay for pneumonia a few years earlier, but also heeding Her Most Wonderfulness's organising voice in my head, I set about gathering wash stuff, pyjamas, underwear, dressing gown, slippers. I was quietly proud of myself, when, off my own bat, I collected her rosary and one of her puzzle books. I would get anything else later.

Reception at A&E took my name and sent me straight through to the ward on the left, not the cubicles that I was used to from my many trips with Arun, but the ones where the serious cases are taken. I asked for directions and was pointed to a curtained off cubicle, where I took a breath, told myself to hold my nerve and stepped inside.

She was tiny, a shrivelled up, dehydrated, raisin-like version of herself and fast asleep. I sat. I had no idea what to do or what to expect, but did not want to disturb her or make things worse, so I found myself leaning further and further forward, staring at her, trying to see whether she was breathing. She was. It was barely perceptible, but I watched each inhalation and exhalation. That was some reassurance, but fear was still piling down on me, so that, when the curtain swished open, I almost fell off the chair.

"Don't worry," said the uniformed medical person. "You're her son, Mark? Is that right? We are rehydrating her and keeping her warm, to get her back to a normal body temp. She was very lucky, but she is already responding encouragingly."

"Is she? She looks so tiny, shrunk," I answered.

"Give her time," she answered in that reassuring, medical manner that is such a gift. "It will take a little while. Do you want to get yourself a drink? We're keeping an eye on her."

I'm a great respecter of calm efficiency and so I accepted her assurance and slipped out to collect a sugar rush and to ring Ranjit with the updates from Amanda and A&E.

"I have no idea what she was doing there, but I'm relieved that I'm going to be able to ask her. Amanda was wonderful and they have things under control here. You know, if she lives through this, I might just kill her myself. I'm sure she's given me a heart attack!"

Back behind her curtain, Moosh was beginning to surface.

Her first words were, "I'm sorry Alistair."

All thoughts of matricide fled, as I half grinned and half sobbed, "You had me so worried. What on Earth were you doing?"

7

Servitude

Nothing could have prepared me for what Moosh shared with me over the next hour and I still struggle to believe it, even now, all these years later.

"I'm so sorry, Alistair, I should have told you what's been happening, but I feel so ashamed," she began.

Every single alarm bell and siren that had been quietening started to clang, shriek and wail in my head.

"Ma, I don't understand. What's happened? Why are you ashamed? Are you in trouble?" I rattled off urgent questions.

"I should have told you, but I was scared of her and was scared that you would be disappointed in me."

The volume of the alarms and sirens ramped up.

"Who? Amanda?" I grappled frantically to get my head round the word her. Apart from her neighbours, and Ranjit and Aly, I did not know any *her*s or *she*s in my mother's life.

At a shake of her head, I was relieved and still puzzled, "No? Not Amanda? Who? Help me, Ma."

"The woman I work for. She is a bad person."

Moosh looked crestfallen, not just shrivelled.

"The woman you work for? Who do you work for? Why are you working? Ma?"

My confusion was mounting with every sentence, every word. Moosh had money, more than enough money. She had my father's pension and her state pension. Everything was paid for: no mortgage to worry about; all bills comfortably covered. She was generous to us and to our children. She had visited her sister in Australia just a few years back. Had she got herself into some sort of trouble that I could not fathom. Had she invested in something, without me knowing?

"Ma, tell me? I promise I won't be disappointed. I just want to help. You've got me worried."

"I keep house for Mrs. Saunders. I clean and I do some gardening for her," she told me.

"Who is Mrs. Saunders? Where did you meet her? At church? Where is her house?" I demanded, unable to keep a burst of anger from my tone.

"I saw an advertisement in the newsagent. I've been worried about running out of money. She lives near the big church in Smethwick. Her address is . . ."

She looked up at me pleadingly. I had not intended to stand over her.

Falteringly, she whispered, "Please. I can't remember her address. It is near the big church."

Unheeding of her distress, more questions boiled out: "Ma, how do you get there? What do you do there? Why is she a bad person?"

I was losing in my effort to regain composure. As soon as Moosh was able to supply an address, I was going to ring the police.

I forced myself to sit and I reached out to hold her hand, which felt feeble and horribly fragile in mine.

"I walk there. And I walk home. The money she pays doesn't cover a taxi or even a bus. She won't let me use her garden tools, so I have to use my hands. If I don't clean to her standard, she screams at me. She even swears. She scares me."

The fear in her eyes cut through me.

"Ma, does she hurt you? Has she hit you?"

"I don't remember."

She looked at her hands. I looked at them, too, trying to see any sign of injury, beyond the dirt beneath her fingernails. There was none.

"I don't remember," she continued. "Maybe. I don't think so."

That gave me no indication whether I could calm down or not. She was clearly terrified, but had she been physically harmed? What could I tell the police? How could I find Mrs. Saunders?

I changed tack, "Ma, if it's the church near the gurdwara in Smethwick, that is over a mile from your house. How do you walk that far? You've been finding walking more difficult. I've been worried with you trying to get to the corner shop, because that is a struggle. How do you do it?"

She looked at me perplexed, with a touch of hurt.

"I manage. Don't you believe me?"

"Of course I believe you, Ma. It's just that I am trying to piece it together. Tell me as much as you can. What do you do in the house?" I prompted.

She began to give me details, "It's one of the big houses. I like the gardening jobs, but there is a lot to do in the house. She is not happy that I'm not strong enough to do the hoovering. I can't move it up and down the stairs. There are a lot of stairs. She threatens me that she will find someone else. I have to do her washing and clean her silver."

"Clean her silver? So, she is quite rich?"

I was trying to gauge where the wealthier properties are located in Smethwick. The name of the church escaped me, but I had friends of friends who lived in a road nearby with larger properties – if I was right about the church. Images of modern-day slavery were flooding my head. How could I have missed this? I fell silent, still holding both of her hands and rubbing with my thumbs, inwardly berating myself. Tears trickled silently towards the pillow. I was caught between calling the police or Sandwell Adult Services. Should I play the card that I had friends high up in Adult Services?

The curtain glided open and the same member of staff entered and stopped abruptly, taking in the scene.

"Is everything OK, Geraldine?" she asked looking first at Moosh and then at me.

Moosh looked at me, mute.

"Please could we speak outside?" I asked, again trying to calm myself.

We stepped out of the cubicle and I kept walking away to create a little distance from Moosh.

When we reached the end of the Assessment Area, I blurted, with far less control than I was hoping for, "I think someone is hurting my mother, or at least terrifying her. She is telling me about things that I have no idea about. I think I need to call the police."

"What has happened?" asked the nurse.

I explained, sharing what Moosh had just told me, trying to leave no detail out.

She nodded, taking in every piece of information and allowing me to finish, before saying, "Mark, we do see this in patients who are dehydrated. Dehydration affects the way the brain works. Geraldine was severely dehydrated when she arrived, which is why we are rehydrating her now."

"But she is very clear about some details; not all, but some. She looks truly terrified," I asserted, trying to emphasise the severity of the situation, as Moosh had explained it to me, and becoming frustrated that I appeared to be failing to communicate my fear.

"That is common in cases of dehydration. The images are very vivid," she said. "Look, let me share this with the doctor, so that he is fully informed, and then he will talk with you. Please don't contact the police just yet. I will get the doctor to come to you and your Mum, as soon as I can. It shouldn't be too long."

I returned to Moosh, trying to have faith in the nurse's hypothesis. I held back from pressing Moosh for further details, only asking how she was feeling, now. She did not return to our conversation, but told me that she was feeling a little better and asked when she could go home.

As promised, a young doctor arrived within minutes.

He explained that he had spoken at length with the nurse, that Mum's readings were improving, the fluids were having a positive effect, but that he wanted to admit Mum for further observation and to allow her to recover fully from the hypothermia and dehydration, with proper medical support.

He then shifted the conversation by offering, "The nurse told me about Geraldine's hallucinations."

"Hallucinations?" I queried.

"Yes," he confirmed, before elaborating, "one of the symptoms or results of dehydration is hallucinations. They can be very vivid and, for the patient, are very real. Geraldine has quite a severe UTI, which has led to dehydration and the onset of what sounds like severe and emotionally disturbing hallucinations. I am very confident that what your mother has shared with you are hallucinations and not something that you need to report to the authorities. Are you comfortable with that?"

"Can we see if Mum speaks about it more, once the hypothermia and the infection and dehydration are fully under control?" I pressed.

"Absolutely. I'll call back later."

Moosh never mentioned Mrs. Saunders ever again, and I never asked. I still can not explain fully what happened inside Moosh's brain, but the feeling that I had failed in my protective role shook me to my core, believing for those tortured minutes that I had not spotted her involvement in servitude and had left her vulnerable.

For a little while, even my rational acceptance that it was all a vivid hallucination did not fully comfort me, and my brain compartmentalised the event as a fall - it's strange how the brain works.

8

The Bed Bath

Moosh gradually recovered and her grip on reality strengthened.

That is not to say it was anywhere near 100%, in fact, it would never be again, but she was much more lucid and able to have meaningful conversations. Encouragingly, she was back to praying, which was always a good sign. She asked me to bring her a wooden hand cross that I had recently bought for her from Liverpool cathedral. It was a perfect size for her to grip in her hand and solid enough that no amount of gripping could break it.

Lucidity and prayerfulness were not strongly connected to reasonable. Moosh frequently confided in me that the nurses were rough and rude. Wanting to be supportive of her and very aware that there are times in every profession when staff fail to operate up to the expected standard, I was careful to observe how she was treated, but also how other patients without visitors around them were being looked after. I did not see one incident of staff acting in any way inappropriately. They were extremely busy. They were run off their feet. They were tired. There never seemed to be enough of them. But, the care they gave was attentive and effective, and often delivered with twinkling humour. I was worried that she was particularly barbed about some of the black staff. She had always brought me up to be respectful, so I was shocked to feel that she might be operating any type of negative, colour filter.

Cantankerousness aside, there were situations where her returning strength and conversation skills combined with ups and downs in lucidity to create situations which had us howling.

One of our collective family howls was on a day that Aly visited with Liam.

By this time, Liam was a punky teenager, experimenting with piercings and adventurous hairstyles that Moosh would have killed me for, but on Liam were pronounced by Moosh to be 'trendsetting'. Liam had also grown into a piss-taker extraordinaire, with 100mph banter that has frequently left me pleading for respite to squeeze at least a tiny breath in. Give him even the most miniscule scintilla of ammunition and he is off and running.

One such scrap appeared while we were sitting with several more than the allowed two visitors per bed, chatting back and forth, when Moosh said, "I'm very worried about the goldfish."

Across the ward from the end of her bed was a well-tended three-foot fish tank. We all turned to check on the ailing goldfish.

Liam, sensing comedy gold, but projecting a veneer of

innocence, enquired, "Which goldfish, Grandma?"

There were no goldfish; it was a tropical aquarium.

"Stop teasing me, Liam," Moosh scolded.

"Where's the goldfish, Ma?" I asked, wanting her to be able to explain.

She waved her finger in a vaguely bottom-of-the-tank direction, "There. The big one. It's not moving. It hasn't moved all day, or yesterday."

Liam loped across to the tank and crouched next to it.

"Here Grandma?" he said, pointing to the corner.

"No. In the middle. Stop teasing!" she gesticulated, in danger of losing her teeth at the onset of giggles.

"Here, Grandma? This big orangey one? The one that is lying very still on the gravel?" he asked, struggling to keep a straight face.

"Yes! That's it!" she warbled, delighted to be proven right.

"The *Plant Pot Fish* is known to prefer the bottom of the tank." Liam narrated in his best David Attenborough tones, with his finger pointing at the ornament placed in front of a clump of artificial weed.

Even Moosh belly-laughed, with her hand in front of her mouth, preventing a denture outage, but she quickly blamed her mistake on the fact that no one had brought her spectacles to the hospital.

To this day, the Plant Pot Fish is fondly recalled, whenever Moosh's grandchildren are reunited.

One of my personal favourites was the day that Her Most Wonderfulness and I arrived to find Moosh positively aquiver and wanting to share her news.

Before we could even sit down, she declared, "I had a bed

bath!"

Before I could point out that this was a good example of her being well cared for, she gushed, "Stuart Grainger came in the night and gave me a bed bath!"

For those of you who are not of an appropriate age (or maybe you have forgotten due to *being* a certain age), Stuart Grainger was an actor in the 1950s and 60s. He was the epitome of suave and debonair, a silver fox and a much-vaunted heart throb. Always cast as a smoothie, he was sure to make a significant portion of any cinema audience swoon. Rather crucially to this tale, he had been dead for over a decade.

"Wow, Stuart Grainger! Giving you a bed bath? Really? That *must* have been a thing!" I humoured her. "You do look very fresh. Did he brush your hair?"

"He did!" she said, patting her head, caught somewhere between beaming and preening.

"And washed your face?" I prodded, enjoying her sparkle.

"He did!" - she almost blushed.

I couldn't stop myself from asking, "Anything else?"

She gave a most unseemly giggle and said, "He went *down there!*"

HMW was struggling to stop herself from shaking with laughter and was in desperate need of an emergency dash to the loo. For me I was caught between, on the one hand the delight of hearing Moosh so animatedly perky and, on the other, that child's place of being horrified at your parents being remotely connected with sex. To see my mother all coquettish and entirely unbecomingly exhilarated following her nocturnal visit from a *hands-on*, 50s heart throb had me flummoxed and I couldn't stop myself.

I had to ask, "How did he get in? Visiting time finishes at eight."

"He volunteers as one of the staff. He wears the proper uniform and everything!" she warbled back, delightedly, before turning to the woman in the next bed and saying, "Doesn't he Doris?"

"Ooooh yes, he does. Stuart Grainger gives a lovely bed bath. Very gentle, but very thorough!" crooned Doris.

To this day, I have never figured out how two women in adjacent hospital beds can have the same fantasy about the enjoyed attentions of a deceased actor, but they were very convinced and just as convincing.

"It will have been a look alike. Actually, they wouldn't have a man giving women bed baths. Would they?" - I was doubting my own argument, even as I said it to Moosh.

"No. It was definitely Stuart Grainger. *Very* gentle!" Doris cooed across.

Whether it was the lingering efficaciousness of the ghostly ablutions administered by Mr. Grainger, I will never know, but Moosh rallied quite quickly and was able to leave hospital by the end of the week and return home. With excellent support from Sandwell's Occupational Therapy service, we had arranged for a number of aids to be installed, grab rails, a wheeled tray, a Zimmer frame and an alarm.

As we were leaving the ward, Moosh asked me to give Doris her wooden hand cross.

When I protested that it was a present from me to her, she countered, "Doris needs it more than me at the moment, don't you think? It will do her good."

Much as I wanted her to keep my gift, it was good to see

her generosity return, if only to counter-balance some of the cantankerousness that she had shown towards a few of the staff. She waved fondly to Doris and her daughter as we passed. Doris had Moosh's cross clasped to her chest.

Years later, when Aly and I were reminiscing about our favourite memories of Moosh, we laughed, as we always do, about Stuart Grainger and the bed bath. It was only then that I learned that, according to Moosh and Doris, Gregory Peck, of *To Kill A Mockingbird* fame, had been volunteering as a doctor on the ward, too. Maybe all hospitals should have ghostly film stars volunteering in different capacities. I wonder whether we could appeal to Liz Taylor to do a couple of days a week at hospitals in Birmingham and Sandwell.

Certainly, the ministrations of Messrs. Grainger and Peck brightened Moosh's stay.

I am surprised we ever got her to leave.

9

The Second Fall

Moosh bounced back remarkably strongly.

She was determined to prove that she could live independently, despite being grateful for the increased frequency of my visits to her house. She capitalised on my detouring via Shakespeare Road on my way home from school by giving demonstrations of her prowess at scooting round the living room and kitchen with her wheeled tray, insisting that I have coffee, so that she could show me how she could bring it to me from the kitchen without me hovering next to her. She Zimmered up and down the garden, pointing out the success of this plant or that, and enthusing about future plans for expanding her beloved shrubbery into the undeveloped distant hinterland of the plot.

Whenever I visited she made sure that I noticed the alarm button that she wore everywhere, hung around her neck. Having at first railed against it, she now viewed the wearing of the alarm pendant as a key weapon in her armoury against my cyclic suggestions that we needed to consider alternatives to her living entirely without support. She had demonstrated to me that she knew how to use it and stated repeatedly that she was happy to do so.

If I pushed too hard in asserting that I'd feel more confident and at ease if she would accept support, she responded testily, "Alistair, I know how to press a button and you know that if I press this button, I will get help. Enough!"

She accepted, with much better grace, my company at all of her appointments at various hospitals. The cocktail of tablets was reviewed and tinkered with to secure maximum impact on her Parkinson's Disease, while also keeping her angina under control. There were assessments and discussions at the Orthopaedic Hospital to improve the functioning of her hip and to ponder when she might require a replacement. She was quite taken with the idea of becoming bionic. She now saw all of the medical support as assistance in her campaign to prolong her independence.

She countered my repeated entreaties to consider coming to live with us with assertions that she hadn't even qualified for a stair lift, because she was so sprightly that she could whizz up and down the steep staircase. She argued, admittedly very rationally (annoyingly so), that if she did not need a stairlift, surely she was still strong enough to live on her own.

She almost weakened, just once, when we took her to see a wonderful six bedroomed, detached house looking down onto Warley Woods golf course, which boasted a truly palatial 'Granny Annexe'. We got so far with the idea that Moosh had agreed to sell her house, pool our finances and make an arrangement for us to pay Aly a portion of the value of Shakespeare Road in the event of Moosh's death, and

Ayesha had excitedly chosen her attic room overlooking the canopy of trees in the woods.

I still find myself looking at that house, a little wistful at the 'what might have beens'.

She was in such a good place that Her Most Wonderfulness and I headed off to Barcelona for a week at Easter, children in tow and feeling reasonably secure.

We were experimenting with city breaks in an attempt to broaden our children's cultural experience. We had introduced them to Paris the previous year, under the thinly disguised pretext of visiting Disneyland, hoping that they would enjoy a city that we had loved since our honeymoon. Barcelona was not our greatest success, given that the children bonded (a positive) over watching Series 10 of *Friends* on repeat for the entire trip and Alex summarised our vacation by declaring that Barcelona looked like a great city, but he'd much prefer to visit with his mates than us. Upon our return, Moosh hooted at hearing this, saying that we should have left the children with her and enjoyed the trip on our own.

At Witsun, we very nearly took her up on her confident offer, when we flew down to Montpellier for a burst of early summer warmth and to be shown the joys of Languedoc. She was back to happily pootling to the local shops and even to catching the bus to West Bromwich; I was almost not worrying, allowing myself to believe that we were enjoying what would be an enduring recovery. Ultimately, however, we played safe and divvied the children out amongst our friends, with Alex staying at home in charge of the house, much to Moosh's huffy indignation and a rebuffed refrain of 'You don't trust me!'s.

We were staggering towards the end of another school year.

July is always busy in any school, but this year we seemed to be running on Flat Out. Unusually for our family, we could not rely on the anticipatory lift of looking forward to heading off somewhere French. Barcelona had been our Big Holiday for the year. To compensate, we were putting together a summer of visiting friends in the UK and reminding ourselves that, as teachers, we should be delighted to be able to look forward to six weeks of comparative rest. Not being entirely persuaded by this line of thought, we were taking any and every opportunity for a little levity that was offered by friends.

We had celebrated my birthday with Moosh just before the weekend, and so were available when friends invited us out for a quick drink on the Sunday evening. Or at least we were available if Moosh could step in and babysit. In truth, there was little actual babysitting involved, as Yeesh was ten years old and needed very little supervision, but we felt safer to be fully covered.

I knew that Moosh would leap at the opportunity to come and spend time at ours and so I rang to ask her whether she was free, and to suggest that I drive round to pick her up, and then pay for a taxi to take her home later in the evening.

There was no answer.

That made sense, as the weather was good enough for her to be out in the garden tending to her plants. I left an answer message, knowing that the likelihood of her picking up the message was slim: she lacked confidence in navigating the technology to retrieve a message, even if she noticed the red-light flashing.

We made alternative arrangements for Yeesh and had a lovely evening out, before getting ourselves ready for the week ahead.

On the Monday evening, after a busy day and an after-school training session, I rang to catch up, but Moosh did not pick up. Again, I looked at the weather outside and was pleased that she would be out with her plants, probably in deep conversation with whatever newly emerging summer flowers had taken her fancy and continuing her never-ending war against infernal bindweed. She would have her alarm hung around her neck. I had heard nothing from the alarm company, so was not concerned.

During the night, however, my brain began to niggle.

I have no idea why that was the case, but, as I stood getting breakfast ready, I decided to take the slight diversion to her house on my way to school. I sped up my wash, shave and shower routine and forced my brain out of the remote-control brain-navigation that gets me to school each day and headed, instead, to Shakespeare Road. I was filled with a blooming sense of foreboding, which peaked as I took the three steps from the car to her door and inserted my key.

Despite the worry that I had woken with, nothing prepared me for the fetid miasma that assaulted me, upon opening the front door. Calling her name, I rushed instantly to the kitchen where she had been found before, but it was empty. I called again but received no answer. I ran up the stairs to her bedroom, passing the bathroom door, which stood slightly ajar, but her room was empty, the curtains open and her bed neatly made and unslept in. The nauseating smell was over-powering, but not coming from her room.

Confused, I rapidly retraced my steps, calling her name as loudly as I dared without wanting to wake the neighbours. Tentatively, I pushed the bathroom door and met resistance. It was then that I heard Moosh: it was the weakest of whimpers. I pushed harder, but the door would open no further.

Concluding that Moosh was lodged behind the door, unable to gain a response to my pleas for her to move or to talk to me, and fearing that I might cause her damage by opening the door against her, I dialled 999.

Biting down on my gag reflex and forcing myself not to give in to the guilty tears that were threatening, I gave the ambulance service the information they needed to come to Moosh's aid. She was clearly conscious and making feeble sounds, both of movement and attempts to speak, but she succeeded at neither.

I slumped outside the door and wept, apologising for not knowing that she was there and for not guessing that something was wrong and for not coming to check up on her. The fact that I could hear her attempting to respond, but failing, only made me cry more. As well as feeling ashamed for not acting sooner, I felt shame that I was embarrassed by the idea of strangers coming into Moosh's house and witnessing her in such a noisome state. Had she been fully aware, she would be appalled too.

In my lifetime, every time that I have needed the emergency services, their response has been rapid and so it proved this time. In minutes, I was beckoning paramedics into the house, apologising for the smell and explaining that I could not reach Moosh in the bathroom and showing them up the stairs.

For the life of me, I can not remember whether they were male or female. What I do remember is their gentle reassurance that they had experienced much worse and the equally gentle suggestion that I wait downstairs to give them room to work their way into the bathroom.

I rang school to let them know that I would not be in and to share what I knew up to that point. I also rang Aly to put her in the picture. She rang back later to let me know that she would make arrangements for Harv to be looked after and then she would head down the motorway to come to see Moosh. Lastly, I rang Ranjit and broke down.

The paramedics alerted me to the fact that they had reached Moosh and that they would be rushing her to A&E. They had eased their way into the bathroom bit by bit, weighing up the risk to Moosh of the force of the door on her body with that of not administering immediate emergency attention. She was alive, but her situation was extremely grave. She was dehydrated, suffering the effects of not eating for approximately sixty hours and horribly weak.

Ranjit arrived and took responsibility for clearing and cleaning the bathroom, a task that I knew was beyond me, not simply for the filth and the smell, but because that small room represented my closest brush with death since visiting my father in the mortuary in Shrewsbury. I could not cope, emotionally, with entering the room and seeing where she had lain.

One of us must have explained to the neighbours what had happened and why the ambulance had come and how they had got on, but I remember none of that. What I knew was that we were about to start the second cycle of trying to retrieve Moosh from the brink of dying. I also knew that I was adamant that Moosh could no longer live alone.

Later, when she was able to speak feebly, Moosh explained that she had fallen, while getting herself ready for bed on Saturday. She had lain on the floor of the bathroom, lodged behind the door, unable to move for almost three days. She had heard the phone ring both times I called, heard my message and had wept that she could not respond.

She was wearing her alarm, but it was pinned beneath her body, rendered useless.

10

Tank

Aly and I, together with Neil and Ranjit, already had a good deal of experience of Moosh's hospital stays.

When Ayesha was due to be delivered, I took Her Most Wonderfulness into Queen Elizabeth Women's Hospital. In the same week Moosh suffered chest pains, which required her own hospitalisation at City Hospital for an angiogram, angioplasty and recovery. She was 67 and full of game, so I think they kept her in hospital to force her to slow down for long enough to give her ticker a much-needed rest.

Each day, I would drive the short (but rush hour affected) journey from school in Handsworth up through Winson Green to Moosh, in her hospital on Dudley Road, for an hour of banter, checking that the expected full recovery was on track and ensuring that she was surrounded by enough treats to keep her in good spirits.

Next, I would head homeward, collecting Arun from Scary Clairy. Most days, Claire had Alex too, filling in for Moosh, who usually looked after him. Once the boys were fed and watered, I would either drop them with HMW's sister, Narinder, or take them to visit their Mom and their beautiful baby sister.

Despite the logistics of Moosh being in one hospital and Her Most Wonderfulness in another, everything went swimmingly. I was riding the crest of a wave of relief, brought on by HMW surviving a full-on asthma attack immediately after Ayesha had been C sectioned out of her. One of the most terrifying scenes I have ever witnessed was the panic of the anaesthetist, who was attending to Ranjit, as he tried to ameliorate her symptoms. However, after that scare, like Moosh, HMW's stay in hospital was primarily to ensure rest, it being her third caesarean. Moosh had had her angioplasty and we had strong assurances from her cardiologist and nurses that she would be fine. As a result, it was just about as stress free as hospital visiting can be: there was no danger.

Roll forward ten years and Moosh's next stay (the one with the joys of the goldfish and the bed bath), had been more stressful. I had experienced that harrowing moment of fear, on the drive to the hospital, that we would lose her, which, although it had been immediately eased by the staff on my arrival, stayed with me. Moosh's evident frailty at that point, both physical and mental, had triggered anxious sibling phone calls about how to ensure that Moosh was safe in her home. With Aly and Neil having moved to the North East, Moosh's extended stay in hospital had necessitated their making numerous trips up and down the motorway. Crucially, though, she had always looked like she would recover.

This new hospital experience was a different beast. There were no reassurances. Even to a non-medical person like me, the gravity of Moosh's situation was starkly clear. There was quiet efficiency and continual, diligent care, but no talk of 'She'll be fine when we . . .' None of that.

Despite having been able to communicate some of what had happened, Moosh was the weakest that I had ever seen a real person be. It was the first time that I truly dwelt in the thought that we might lose her. It was the first time that I thought that it might be better for her if she did not pull through, so desperately diminished and feeble was she, as I watched her struggling to hold on to life. It was the first time that Moosh had ever expressed to me that she believed her own death might be imminent and requested that the Last Rites be administered to her.

I consulted the sister on the ward, who agreed that this was a sensible step for a person in Moosh's condition, but suggested that the need was not immediate, so I could arrange for her priest to visit the next day.

Unheeding of the sister's assurance, her agreement that it might be wise to arrange for the Last Rites to be given freaked me into deviating from Moosh's wishes that I call her church, the Oratory. I did not know the clergy there. In truth, there was only one church in the whole of Birmingham where I could claim to know any of the clergy, but, fortuitously, it happened to be St. Patrick's, directly across the Dudley Road from the main entrance of the hospital.

Through a friend from teacher training college, I knew that, by wonderful coincidence, Canon Piercy was now parish priest at St. Pat's. He had been the bursar from my old boarding school and would forever in my mind be known as *Tank*. It was somehow fitting for me that Tank should be the one to tend to Moosh, given the regard that they had for one another when I was a boy. Making my call to him brought back vivid memories of bouncing along rural North Staffordshire roads in his lovingly maintained workhorse of a Morris Minor, with Tank, his aged mother and Moosh, as he delivered us to Uttoxeter station.

Having listened, as I explained to him who I was, and Moosh's situation, I was taken aback by his immediate remembrance of both she and I.

His quiet pledge of, "I will be there first thing tomorrow, Mark," brought a much-needed smile to my face for three reasons.

Crucially, I had managed to secure a visit from a priest. Secondly, I thought it would be lovely for Moosh to meet Tank again, after thirty years, despite the circumstances. Far less importantly, it was the first time in either of our lives that he had not called me *Lanyon*, as he would have done at school, or *108*, which he used to scribe with an ancient, scratchy nib onto the fabric of every item of sports clothing that I purchased from him.

With school being so demanding and Aly uncertain when she could get down from Loftus, neither of us was in attendance when Canon Piercy visited Moosh. When he phoned me to let me know that he had done the deed, his pleasure at being reacquainted with Moosh was a world away from the rather diffident man I remembered. The gentleness of his promise that he would keep Moosh in his prayers was entire galaxies away from the legendary rugby playing hardman, scourge of opposition teams, which some said was the reason he was called Tank. I was touched and grateful, but still terrified. To me the act sharply signified the fraying thread of Moosh's mortality.

When I visited that evening, despite still being physically weak, Moosh was visibly, spiritually uplifted and so bursting to share news of seeing Canon Piercy that she quickly forgave me for not ringing the Oratory.

She was in good humour for the first time since her emergency admission, repeatedly smilingly saying, "What a lovely man. Such twinkly eyes." (Tank not me)

When Moosh then suddenly switched direction and asked me whether I thought that she had been a good Mum, I was still caught up in the spark of levity and the buoyant emotions fostered by Tank's visit. I gave an off the cuff, jocular response and received a featherlight punch on my arm for my playful impertinence.

To my surprise, as I headed across the car park to start my drive home, I met Alyson coming the other way with her friend from home, Marie, who was armed with a box of doughnuts.

As we all hugged, I filled Aly in on Tank's visit and Moosh's better spirits but continued fragility and regaled them with my witty answer to Moosh, "It's not too late to start trying, what with you wanting the best seat in Heaven!"

Suddenly mindful that I hardly knew Marie, I apologised for the Lanyon humour.

Marie laughed, "No. Fair play. Hasn't Moosh been threatening to die?"

As I turned right onto Dudley Road, I passed St. Patrick's on the left and called out a silent message of gratitude to Tank, proud that I had fulfilled Moosh's wishes and hoping that the uplift in her spirits would morph into an improvement in her physical condition.

Little did I know what I had left Alyson and Marie to walk in to.

11

The Golden Son List

Something gave Moosh renewed strength.

Either Tank's visit and the Last Rites were efficacious in unexpected ways, or my quip unintentionally opened a sore, but between my leaving and Aly arriving with Marie, Moosh was in high dudgeon. She had not known that Aly would be visiting, but it was as if she was waiting for her, ready to attack. Or maybe she would have done the same to whoever had visited her next.

What Aly described to me was a Moosh that I still struggle to recognise.

As I have said, our experiences of being her children were sometimes, possibly even frequently, unrecognisably different. I struggle to remember a single time in my life when Moosh was unkind or nasty to me. While I have heard her make negative comments about others, passersby, strangers, people on television, and witnessed her being awkward, bordering on belligerent with Ranjit, it was Alyson who caught the negative opposites to the positivity that was showered on me.

I never understood it and I regret that I did little to question or change it, although, in my defence, the worst excesses never occurred in my presence. They were reported to me, often years later.

As soon as Aly and Marie had seated themselves, Moosh instructed Aly to find some paper and a pen. When this was done, Moosh told Aly that she was to write for her. Over the next almost two hours, while Marie listened with increasing incredulity, Moosh dictated an exhaustive list of my positive attributes.

The only interruption to Moosh's flow and Aly's scribing was the woman in the next bed, who had spied Marie's doughnut offering. After looking at them covetously for several minutes, she tentatively asked Marie for one.

Marie, being Marie, was in the act of passing one across when Moosh snapped, tartly, "No! They are mine!"

Shocked by Moosh's affronted stance and the rudeness of her tone, Marie mutely apologised to the neighbour and withdrew her hand. For the remainder of the visit, Marie sat silently in witness to Aly being made to transcribe her brother's strengths, until she cried at the injustice, unable to believe what she had observed. Unmoved or un-noticing, Moosh completed her dictation.

In spite of the hurt that Aly felt, before they left, she leant over the rail of Moosh's bed to hug her and kiss her. Being just over five feet tall, Aly struggled to fully reach Moosh, but stretched to the limits of her tendons to ensure that she was at her very tallest.

When I arrived the next day, Moosh's mood was somewhere

between disgruntled and pained. My first instinct was that her strength was dipping, but I was sorely mistaken: she was quietly seething.

To my enquiry as to what was troubling her, she insisted that Aly had left the previous evening without saying, "Goodbye."

Entirely innocent of any knowledge of what had taken place the night before, I thought it best to give Aly a call to let her know what Moosh had told me. I stepped out of the ward and rang her.

"That's so unfair, Al-"

Aly began to answer, before dissolving into gulping sobs on the other end of the line.

For several minutes, I listened to her tears until she was able to compose herself and continue, "Al, I couldn't actually speak when we were leaving. If I had tried to say anything, I think I would have done exactly what I've just done and make a complete show of myself on the ward."

There was another lachrymose pause before Aly recounted what had taken place the night before, concluding, "I have Moosh's list for you. It must be nice being you. Being adored."

Before I could respond, she blurted, "Sorry! That was unnecessary - it's not your fault. Sorry Al."

She must have been visualising the scene again, because she astonished me by starting to laugh.

"You should have seen that poor, bloody woman in the next bed! She was mortified, poor cow! I won't be able to face her next time I come!"

I laughed along with her, trying to pull her up out the sorrow in her voice, to assuage the pain just a little, but her tone was bleak when she said, "Maybe I shouldn't come for a while, Al. It's you she wants."

Appalled, I said, "Let me call you back in a few minutes."

I managed not to storm back into the ward. Nor did I raise my voice to Moosh. She was still my Mum. However, in the sternest son to mother voice that I thought I could use, while causing least disturbance to staff and patients, I scolded Moosh in no uncertain terms, letting her know that I had left Aly in tears on the phone and telling her what had been reported to me about the previous evening.

To her credit, she was immediately remorseful, "Oh no, I only wanted for you to know how much I love you. I was trying to show you that I *am* a good mother."

"And what about Aly's feelings? Did you not think of them? Didn't you realise how it would look to her?"

At my admonishment, she looked crestfallen and, at my suggestion that we ring Aly to try to put things right, she readily agreed.

I am not sure what I could have done if she hadn't, but Aly allowed me to put Moosh on the phone and heard her apology. To my ears, the apology was sincere, although I do not believe that it reached Aly's heart, leaving another open wound alongside multiple scars inflicted by four decades of grievances.

Consoling myself that I had tried to heal the rift quickly, and knowing that I hadn't at all, I focussed instead on spending time with Moosh, keeping her talking, remembering Tank's mother and asking whether she needed me to bring anything else for her. Gradually her equilibrium returned, although she still looked as if a decent draft would whisk her away. If

I knew how to lay a bet, I would have gambled large on her not having much life remaining.

Caught somewhere between fearing the worst, and fearing that the worst might actually be the best thing for her, and because I guessed that it was important to her, I returned to the answer that I was horribly certain had been the catalyst to all of this hurt, or at least this chapter of it: "Ma, I think you have been a wonderful Mum. To Ranjit and me and to all of your grandchildren you have been generous, kind and loving. I would not be who I am without the things you have done for me and the way you raised me. I wish I knew what it was with you and Aly, but I can't pretend to."

Moosh reached wordlessly for my hand with her gnarly one and we sat.

As I left, hoping that Moosh would still be there when I next came back, my eye fell on the doughnut-seeking neighbour, who herself looked at death's door and thought to myself that she could have done with one of those.

At some point, Aly did actually give me Moosh's list, in her flowery, flowing script. I never could bring myself to read it, knowing the pain that had gone into the recording of it, its emotional cost. However, I did keep it. It is somewhere safe.

Perhaps, one day, I will read it, when all of the hurt is gone. After all, they are Moosh's words - to me.

But that time hasn't arrived yet.

12

No Resuscitation

After the insensitivity of Moosh's valedictory list, I was stunned by Aly's brilliance at staying in contact with the hospital.

She was soon on first name terms with almost every member of the medical team attending to Moosh. While I tend to baulk at being seen as a nuisance, Aly, rightly, insistently sought daily updates on Moosh's condition. If information had been promised but not given, or if she had been told that a change was expected or a test was being carried out, she would ring more frequently.

By the following Thursday, nine days after Moosh's admission, Aly's pooling of information had convinced her that Moosh's condition was becoming critical and she asked Liam's girlfriend, Jess, to drive down to the Midlands with her. Her reading of the situation and the timing of her visit proved to be perfect, as, on her arrival, she found Moosh unresponsive and the medical staff concerned.

She was immediately taken to an adjacent office to be

updated and her views sought. From there, she rang me, simply letting me know that she was in Birmingham and asking me to meet her at the hospital, where she would fill me in on what she had been told.

I arrived from school, mind already somewhat wired from a day of school self-evaluation and action planning for the new year that would start in September, and knowing that my expectation of myself meant that I would return to school by 6:00pm for the Year 6 Leavers' Production, despite no one at school feeling that I should. I had psyched myself up for whatever news there was regarding Moosh's condition, but not for drama. I expected Aly and I to be tearful, but was not ready for alarums.

Given the calm with which she had managed to speak to me on the phone, I was entirely unprepared for the tenterhooks I found Aly on, or her rapid-fire, opening gambit of, "No resus or resus, what do you think? We must state our wishes! Today!"

"What? What is resus? No resus? What is that?" I was bemused and deteriorating from wired to garbled in milliseconds. I had vague recollections of the word *resus* from medical dramas, but I'm not a big fan of those given the blood and their propensity for people dying.

Slowing down for my benefit, Aly named a nurse or a doctor that she had been speaking to, saying, "They've said that Moosh is still very weak and that it is likely that, at some point soon, a situation will arise in which they will need to resuscitate her. Given her frailty, there is the question of whether that is in her best interests and what she would want, but she is not conscious to give that information, so we must decide."

She took a quick breath, before adding, "Now."

"Now? Now what?" I was not keeping up.

"Al, we have to tell them today. Like *now*."

Aly's answer forced the surfacing of unwanted comprehension of this unanticipated level of drama. I was instantly tipped into a world of ethical debate that I did not want to embrace and was most certainly not ready to consider.

"They need us to decide whether they fight to keep her alive or let her go gently? Is that where we are at? We are deciding whether she would want to live or die? Am I right?" I asked.

Obviously, it wasn't Alyson's fault, but I am certain that I was unfairly terse.

She nodded.

Neither she nor I are sure where she went next, but I remember with absolute clarity, sitting on one of those inhospitably hard chairs in the corridor, almost serene in the surrealness of it all. It was the only time in my life in which I have knowingly had the power to make a life or death decision, yet here I was in a dreamlike state of calm as I focused on hearing Moosh's voice inside my head, or my heart, or my soul.

The thing that holds those minutes in such sharp focus for me, is that I became aware of a parent of one of our Year 6 children, who would be in that evening's performance, sitting in the chair one down from me. She acknowledged me and said that she was seeing her mother and I told her the same. A part of me needed to share what I had to decide, but professional boundaries and good sense stopped me in time. I wished her mother well, said that I would catch up with her at school and excused myself as I went in search of the chapel.

As I walked the long corridor of the hospital, I already knew my thoughts. I had probably known them for years. They were ingrained in the fabric of who I am, but I needed solitude to be sure of myself and of the words I would say to Aly. I was sure that Moosh would agree. Thankfully the chapel was both open, as I expected, and empty, as I hoped, leaving me free to cry out my feelings, before returning to search for Aly.

She was sitting with Moosh.

Moosh was the same, unconscious and hanging on a thread.

Aly looked up at me and said, "You've decided, haven't you?"

"Yes, but it is a decision for both of us." I insisted.

"I know, but you are my big brother, so what have you decided?" she pushed.

"I think that Moosh wants to be with Dad. I think that given the choice between being kept alive to live a life of frailty and further deterioration, or passing away, gracefully, now, she would go with Dad," I said. "But I have to be clear, Aly, that my own thoughts on quality of life come into this. I have always felt that we should be able to choose an out, if our chances of a dignified life are jeopardised. If it were me in Moosh's position, I would want to be able to click the off switch or know that someone I loved would do it for me. I think she hates that her body is letting her down and that she would want to be released."

Chin quivering, Aly reached out for my hand, "You've said it better than me, but that it is what I think too. I love you, Al."

"I love you too, Aly," I answered, "but it's all a bit shit this, isn't it? I'm not sure that I signed up to be a grown up."

"Too fucking right, it is. Shit, I mean!" she said, quivering giving way to tearfulness. "And you'll never be a grown up. Not really. Well, only when you have to be. Don't you need to be grown up now and go to your kids' Leavers' Production?"

"I should," I agreed, "but we had better let the staff know what we have decided."

Capitalising on her relationship with the nurses, Aly asked for the doctor to come as soon as possible. He arrived in minutes and I found myself stating, calmly and clearly, that, should Moosh reach a point where resuscitation was necessary, our wishes were that it would be withheld.

And there it was: the single most difficult decision I have ever had to make.

Aly assured me that she would take care of any further conversations with the doctor needed that night and urged me to go back for the production at school. So, with a squeeze of Aly's hand and a benedictory placing of my hand on Moosh's head, I found myself walking out of the ward, donning my imaginary Superman pants, tunelessly humming the theme tune from the film in my mind and heading back to work.

As always, the children were wonderful, their parents were proud and I, already well known for being emotional in school assemblies, tried hard to hold myself together.

I explained my quavering voice by saying, "I came back

83

from visiting my Mum in hospital, so that I could be with the children for their production and I'm so very pleased that I did. I wouldn't have missed it for the world."

Then I blubbed.

Our school was like that, very much 'heart on your sleeve'.

Afterwards, as they went home, ten and eleven-year-old children came over to say, "Sir, I hope that your Mom will be OK. Thinking of you."

And parents came over to break professional boundaries and give me a hug.

As I drove home, wrung out, the enormity of our decision threatened to swamp me.

13

Confession

To this day, Aly swears that some small part of Moosh must have been aware of that bedside conversation with her doctor.

Having remained with Moosh, Aly is certain that, maybe only subliminally, she heard me stipulate no resuscitation. She is adamant that it was from that moment that Moosh first rallied haltingly, then turned back from her Heavenward path and ultimately revived, some of her strength returning, together with an even greater portion of her feistiness.

Aly continued to stay with her, until she was assured that Moosh was no longer at death's door and that she was out of immediate danger, which was long enough for Moosh to declare the hospital food inedible and to demand to know when she would be going home.

To stop me worrying and to give me half a chance of getting a night's sleep, Aly rang me after the Leavers' Production.

Her relief was almost tangible as she reported, "She's come back to life, Al. Those poor nurses are in for a bit more running around."

Given the lateness of her wait at the hospital and her depleted emotional reserves, Aly had decided not to attempt the drive home, crashing instead at Moosh's house and fuelling up on pizza and coffee.

Next day, pleading extenuating circumstances, she managed to wangle a free pass outside visiting hours to be able to go see Moosh before her journey back to Loftus. She wangled me one too, so I raced out of school, stealing an hour after the end of year Y6 Graduation, and we met at the hospital. It felt a little naughty to be a) out of school and b) the only visitors on the ward, but I much preferred the ward that way: quiet and almost peaceful with the staff left to do their jobs.

One of Aly's allies on the staff freed herself to talk to us about what the future held, as we were both keen to know when Moosh would be released; what we should expect; what we would need to arrange; and who we could look to for support.

Being much more in the loop of conversation with the team on the ward and having a yen for all things medical, Aly was of the understanding that, even if she continued her revival, the likelihood was that Moosh would need an extended period of monitoring and medical care, which could only happen in hospital. I expressed what I knew to be true, that Moosh would want to be out, causing mayhem in the wider world.

Aly was right. I knew that she was. I even agreed with her, but I also knew, selfishly, that if Moosh was kept in hospital, it would fall to me to tell her. We both looked to the nurse, part of my mind going through the whole 'You know you'regetting old, when the nurses look young' routine.

I hoped that it didn't show on my face as she explained, "Knowing Geraldine, I'm sure you are right, Mark, that she will want to be going home. She is stronger than she was yesterday, and she is out of any immediate danger, but she is a very long way from being strong enough to be released."

Both Aly and I gave each other a smile.

I'm not sure what I looked like, but a few years fell away from Aly's face, before the nurse, who I was now looking on very kindly, continued, "But she will need to stay in hospital until we can make her safe and address her needs, as far as we are able. We are arranging for her to be transferred to Sheldon Block, where we care for our longer-stay patients. In time, the staff there will work with you to identify what Geraldine will need in the longer term, but the first priority will be to stabilise her and rebuild her strength."

I groaned and Aly gurned gleefully, quickly explaining to the nurse that it wasn't Moosh's further incarceration that she was grinning at, but the knowledge that it would be me who had to tell our mother. Winning even more Brownie Points from me, the young nurse offered for one of the medical staff to explain the plan to her, but I told her that, despite my sister's entirely inappropriate mirth and heartless hilarity, I agreed that the news would be better coming from me.

If you can do such a thing in a vehicle, Aly scuttled North, mightily relieved at Moosh's resurgence but still chuckling at my discomfort. I headed back to school for the happy chaos of the last day of the academic year activities, to gather my thoughts internally, as outwardly we said goodbye to the children and their parents for the summer and sent the staff off for a much needed rest.

I mulled and pondered and prevaricated, carefully marshalling my arguments and going over my wording, but, ultimately, I knew that I had to bite the proverbial bullet and just tell Moosh. I like to think that it was my diligent preparation that did the trick, but I was more than slightly stunned that Moosh took the news rather better than I expected. I had stressed the need for her strength to return and she fully agreed that she still felt weak, despite being very grateful to be alive.

Suffused with the warm glow of my success, I had one more thought burrowing away uncomfortably in my mind, a nagging doubt that I needed to share.

Feeling much like my pre-teen self, entering the confessional at church, I said, "Ma, when you were very ill, yesterday, Aly was told that you might not last the day. She was told that we must decide whether you should be resuscitated, if the need arose. She asked me to come, so that we could decide what we should do. I felt certain that you would want to be with Dad and so I told the doctor not to try to resuscitate you. Was that the right thing to do? Was that what you wanted?"

Moosh, still tiny and delicate, appeared to look inward, lost in some internal conversation, before a radiant smile blossomed on her face, and in barely a whisper she said, "You are right, Alistair, I do miss Daddy, but I believe that God will take me only when he wants me. I would have asked to be resuscitated."

I was mortified.

Moosh saw tears spring to my eyes.

I had not realised that I had reached for her hand, but I felt hers squeeze mine.

"Ma, I would have let you go. You could have died. I was so sure. I'm so sorry!"

Utterly devastated, I was barely damming the flood inside.

Moosh squeezed again, "I'm proud of you. You took responsibility. Thank you. If God wanted me, he would have taken me. I'm still here with you, so it wasn't my time."

Transformed from a forty-three-year-old man, an experienced head teacher always willing to make difficult decisions, to a mother's son crushingly aware of having weighed up the options and made an enormous error of judgement, I was aghast. Moosh's sincere words were insufficient to console me and the tears brimmed over.

She continued the gentle reassurance of her grip, allowing me to wrestle with the guilt I felt at being willing to let her go, to withhold the attempt to save her. The knowledge that I had thought so carefully, sought to hear her voice and still been entirely wrong, filled me with horror and, worse, self-loathing. I accused myself of being selfish and wanting my mother dead.

Finally, I returned the clasp of her hand and repeated, "I'm just so sorry."

There was little more that I could say.

I rarely get out-of-control drunk.

I am far too fearful of following in my Dad's drink-drenched footsteps and of repeating the life threatened ambulance trip of my 21st birthday, when I had temporarily stopped breathing. Where Dad had been a maudlin drunk, I was more of an accident-prone disaster waiting to happen, which I generally made certain to avoid, almost always managing to stay on the entertaining side of stupidly tipsy.

That night, however, with The Dog full of teachers celebrating freedom, I allowed myself to get head-poundingly drunk, until the remorse was lost in the haze.

The next morning was far from pretty, other than being pretty grim. Having noisily voided my own stomach in the night, I hungrily ingested the only hangover cure that works for me, a greasy full English breakfast with Her Most Wonderfulness's chilli baked beans.

Then I gave myself a strict talking to, coupled with a hefty kick up the bum and decided that it was time for me to stop feeling sorry for myself: Moosh needed me.

14

Geriatrics!

In the first week of the summer holiday, as Moosh was transferred to Sheldon Block, little could we have guessed that she would be there for the entire summer and then for the first half of the next term, three months all told.

The first day was dreadful and, in many ways, it would be indicative of her entire stay.

I was not actually with her when she was moved. I have no idea how it happens, whether the bed is pushed along corridors and taken down in one lift and across the hospital grounds, before ascending in another lift. What I do know is that when I arrived, much preferring the new building and grateful for its proximity to the car park, it was to find a small explosion waiting to detonate.

"Old people!" she hissed. "They've put me with a room full of old people! Geriatrics! Dozens of them! Look!"

Obediently, I did indeed scan around the open-ended room that made up the section of the ward to which she had been allocated, trying not to stare. Reluctantly, I registered very clearly that Moosh made a very valid point. She was exaggerating when she claimed 'dozens', but the age demographic of the ten women in the ward was certainly upward of 70. In my PC way, I would, even then, have hesitated to explicitly describe them as "old" but they were almost uniformly tired looking and ashen in pallor. The only other person whose skin did not have a greyish tinge, looked disconcertingly jaundiced.

"We are all here waiting to die!"

Her less than subtle whisper brought me sharply back to her with an alarmed, "Shhhh, Ma!"

I was so embarrassed that I almost covered her mouth, while trying to ascertain whether her neighbours had heard her.

Within a week, Ranjit, myself and the children had developed a fluid timetable of visits, navigating around other commitments and rotating our visit schedule to make sure that Moosh never passed a day without at least one of us spending an hour with her. Aly and the Loftus crew supplemented our rota, when Harv's needs and time allowed.

Within the fluidity of the timetable, each visit was soul-strippingly routine. Gather together bag of that day's things for Moosh. Park car as close to Sheldon Block as possible. Take lift to the 5th floor. Alcohol hand wash on the way in. Affix grin to face. Deliver treats. Restock Moosh's bedside cupboard. Check for what was needed on next visit. Collect laundry. Hour of chat (news from the outside world, opinions formed from her newspaper reading, her account of other patients' ups and downs, and her gripes – always, always gripes). Alcohol hand wash on the way out. I could do the entire visit right now, as I write, so programmed did I become that summer.

I even reached the point where I recognised other visitors, so often did we arrive and leave at the same time, nodding greetings to one another and asking after each other's loved ones, encouraging, commiserating, celebrating or offering condolences as appropriate.

When one of the fathers from school was admitted to a ward somewhere else in the same building, suffering the after-effects of a severe stroke, he and I would regularly meet in the foyer downstairs and chat, I asking after his children (who were still on school holiday) and he offering prayers for Moosh.

The person who never ever settled into the routine was Moosh.

She grizzled about the food, often loudly. She complained about her neighbours, thankfully less loudly, but often with gestures, flicks of the head and scowls. Sometimes I had to stop myself from laughing, because she often reminded me of those vintage Les Dawson and Roy Barraclough comedy sketches of the cheerfully moaning old housewives.

In her weird, twitching-faced code she managed to convey who snored loudest, who suffered from continual, pungent flatulence, who shouted at the nurses in the night and who had wet their bed, something that appalled her.

She was genuinely fearful of The Walkers, those patients who roamed in the night, sometimes getting lost, sometimes trying to get out of the ward. Especially alarming for her were the male Walkers, who would come to her female section and stand and stare.

More than anything she was afraid of dying in that building. A fear that was magnified when the jaundiced looking woman in the bed opposite her passed away during the night. The flurry of activity, as emergency care was given, behind curtains rapidly swished closed, unnerved her and she pleaded through silent tears to be taken home.

I could not take her home, but I could take her out of the ward.

At first, we took to visiting a large room towards the end of the ward, away from her section. Although much of it was taken up with spare chairs, and a selection of wheelchairs and walking frames, it was possible to shift furniture around to create a space to sit in privacy, not surrounded by other patients and their families.

Later, I asked permission to take her out into the grounds, when the weather was clement. I had found an enclosed garden and she loved it. Just the fresh air and being outside would have been sufficient, but to have plants to look at and touch and name and talk about was a real boon. Even though, after decades of being her son, I had a fairly decent knowledge of plants, she relished this unexpected opportunity to teach me about the ones that we found in that garden. Even though I recognised many of the plants, I never let on, so that she could have the joy of instructing me, mining her encyclopaedic knowledge.

On those escapes from the ward, away from others' ears, Moosh and I refound our ability to engage in lengthy conversations. Although we were assured by the medical staff that she was becoming stronger and were encouraged by positive talk of her leaving hospital before the end of the year, the enforced recognition of Moosh's mortality, and how close we had come to losing her this time, accentuated my desire to get to know her even better. I had always felt close to her, but, as is often the way, I had fallen into the habit of taking her for granted. Not so much what she did for us, I was always grateful for that, but that childlike assumption that she was infinite and would always be around.

So, we talked.

She relished those conversations, but deep down, I knew that what she enjoyed most was having me all to herself.

One sunny day, I wheeled her out to our bit of garden, wrapped in a blanket against a slight chill that belied the sun's brightness. As we expected, the garden was all ours.

Without having planned to, I found myself asking her whether she had found happiness in her life. I knew that her early years had been blighted with separation from first her parents and then her older sister, Marguerite, but I knew also that there had been love and friendships that she valued and adventures that she had been on. There had been that epic trip, just a few years earlier, when she had travelled to the other side of the globe to spend a fortnight with Marguerite in Adelaide.

Her answer gave me pause for thought, when, after reflecting inwardly for some time, she said, "Yes. I have been happy, most especially for the last seventeen years."

My first reaction was to be delighted that she could identify herself as having experienced happiness.

My second was to calculate backwards seventeen years and I gasped, "Dad passed away nineteen years ago!"

She looked at me quietly, allowing that to sit between us,

my mind whirring until I realised: "Alex was born seventeen years ago! Grandchildren!"

It was true. Just as Her Most Wonderfulness has done years later, Moosh fell entirely in love, when her grandchildren came along. It was that pure adoration that is free of all of the worry and responsibility associated with parenthood. Aly's children and ours had benefitted enormously from that love, but sitting in that garden, I was delighted to be reminded that Moosh had done too. In that moment, her radiance did not come from the sun shining down on her, but from a reservoir of memories and love harboured and cherished deep within, and it was wonderful to behold.

Although that is the conversation that is indelible in my memories, we went out as often as her strength and the weather allowed and the conversations lifted her. At the end of them, however, we still had to go back to a ward full of what Moosh had decided was, 'Us dodderers, waiting to die'.

We needed to get her out of there!

15

Up North

Rather brilliantly, we did not need to push hard.

The medical team around Moosh were pleased with her progress and were happy to discuss with us plans for her future care. It was very clear to everyone that Moosh would never again be able to live entirely independently. I was a little taken aback that Moosh accepted this, but she did - reluctantly. After two near misses, she recognised that it would not be prudent to tempt fate by risking another.

Given the green light by Moosh's acceptance, back at home Ranjit and I mulled and pondered and deliberated round and round, backwards and forwards, exploring options for Moosh. Was it time to revisit the option of buying a bigger house and have Moosh come to live with us? Clearly, it would have its challenges with our jobs and the children's lives to be taken into account, but it *was* one option.

We felt certain that Moosh would dismiss the idea of a care home or even sheltered housing, because she had always held a pursed-lipped dislike of the very notion of the involving of outsiders in her life, magnified enormously by her lengthy stay in hospital. We were clear that the medical support that she was receiving should still be accessible, so a local option was best.

I met up with Aly on one of her visits, keen to hear her take on the way forward and to share where Ranjit and I had reached in our discussions.

"I want Mum to come to live with us."

That was Aly's opener.

Just to be clear, in case I had not understood, she continued, "In Loftus."

I must have looked entertaining, because Alyson laughed, perhaps at my astonishment, but more likely, at my outright disbelief. Her laughter was pencil-thin and brittle.

"I've surprised you, haven't I? I've surprised myself to be honest."

"After everything?" I blurted. "After you were so hurt by her? That night, with the list and Marie? And the way you two are?"

"I know," Aly conceded. "She does my head in, but she's my Mum and I love her. I want to do this."

"But Harv?" I asked.

Harv required 100% of Aly, or close to it. Since his diagnosis with autism, Aly had built her life around researching the autism spectrum and analysing Harvey's needs and responding to them. She also worked with other families with autistic youngsters, having them come to stay at her home where she would assess the children and develop programmes for the families to implement.

"That's precisely why I can do it, when you can't," she

replied.

"I am already at home with Harv. I have to be there, but Harv doesn't need me every second of every day. As long as he has the things he needs and things he wants, he is happy. And I have time on my hands.

"You, on the other hand, have no time. You are focussed on school and Moosh already stops you doing that now and she's not even living with you. Were you thinking of having her live with you? Buying the big house?"

"We have talked about it, yes," I admitted.

"You know that won't work," Aly stated. "You are too committed to work and you love it, plus you've done the 'emotional capacity maths' in the past and you know that it would be stretching yourselves too far and way too thin.

"But more to the point, this is my time. I want to do this. I want to be able to do it for Mum. And I want to be able to do it for me. I think it will help us. Both of us."

Hearing the need, I was reluctant to raise obstacles, but felt that I had to moot, "Aly, I get that. It is brave and laudable, but all of her support has been here. Quite apart from all of her Parkinson's support, she's also being checked out for a hip replacement and –"

"And they can replace hips up there," Aly laughed, still thinly, wearily. "And we dispensed with gas lighting years ago. We do have hospitals Up North, too.

"Everything that is being done for her down here can be done where we are. I can project-manage all of that with minimal impact on our lives, whereas you have to take time out of work or fit things into your holidays. It would be better, Al."

She was making plausibly good sense. If she and Moosh

could modify the dynamics of their relationship, and if Aly could, indeed, balance caring for Harv with caring for Moosh, it might work. They had the physical space in their house, right down to a large, accessible, ground floor bathroom, right next to a reception room that could be given over to Moosh. And, apparently, there were indeed, 'hospitals Up North'. But –

"Aly, what if it doesn't work? What if it is too much, or if it goes wrong?" I pressed, wanting to offer her an escape route.

"Then we rethink. We think about a care home, *then*. But not *now*."

She was determined, concluding her pitch with, "I have to do this. I believe that I can."

"And your back?" I queried. "It's always been iffy."

I hated myself for voicing another obstacle that I did not want to pose, but felt should be considered. Aly had suffered from sciatica-type back pains and spasms for much of her adult life.

In for a penny, in for a pound, I finished, "And you're not getting any younger."

"Fuck off, smart arse!"

Finally, she was laughing more fully, "Neil and Liam will be around at least some of the time to lift and carry. I will look at accessing support through social services. If I need to bring in a carer to work alongside me, I will. I think we have those Up North too, you know."

"If Moosh lets you." I pointed out, instantly stifling the lighter tone that I had been trying to induce.

"Yes." Aly nodded. "There is that bit. What Mum will allow. But we will find a way."

And that was how the plan was hatched.

"Brave," offered Ranjit, when I told her. "Very brave of Aly, but fair play to her for stepping up. That's huge. What will Geraldine say?"

I had no idea what to expect, none of us did, but Moosh delighted us all by accepting Aly's offer with genuine gratitude and, when she and I talked, she was full of excitement at the idea of living in Loftus with Aly and her family, and seeing Liam and Harvey grow up at close quarters.

Feeling that I had to plant a seed, I cautioned Moosh, "You will be kind won't you, Ma? This is huge for Alyson. She really wants to make this work for you, for both of you. You will need to help her by listening. I can't pretend that I have ever understood the two of you, but you will need to do your part in making this work."

Moosh bridled briefly at my presumption, but quickly supressed any bite back that might have been percolating, "I will be very well behaved. I promise."

As I sealed our pact with a hug, she mumbled on my shoulder, "You are going to visit me, aren't you?"

"Maybe," I chuckled, before she pinched me. "Of course I will. Often. And I'll bring you back here for holidays to see the children. I promise. And if you do behave, I might even take you to the Oratory."

In late October, Neil and Aly moved Moosh to Woodlands, ready to rearrange their lives. They took favourite pieces of furniture from Shakespeare Road together with beloved belongings and ornaments to create a new home for her, her final home. Aly's hope was that Moosh would live her last years there and, when the time was right, pass away peacefully in the bosom of her family.

We were all delighted that Moosh was free, admittedly diminished and much more fragile, but away from hospital and back out in the world, ready to live.

III

Part Three

Woodlands
October 2006

16

Sheffield

With Moosh's move north to Loftus, my hate-love relationship with the M1 motorway began.

I had always found the journey to Aly and Neil's fairly benign, with the bonus of some stunning scenery, particularly the miles that are reached after skirting round Leeds. Ordinarily, I would expect to complete the 200 mile trip in around three hours, door to door.

Moosh had been installed at Woodlands, Aly and Neil's home, for a fortnight, when I made my first planned visit. Hoping to spend at least part of the weekend back at home with Ranjit and the children, I had arranged to leave school at the end of Friday lunchtime. With the blessing of Elaine, my deputy, I arrived at school at Stupid O'clock, so that I had already put in three hours before the children arrived just before 9:00am, and four more before I left at 1:00pm. She agreed to take care of business and attend to any of the multitude of disasters that only ever seem to happen on a Friday afternoon.

Logic told me that traffic might be busy on a Friday afternoon and I was determined to beat the Leeds rush hour, so it was with unseemly haste and enormous gratitude that I whisked past the school office, with loud cries of 'Lots of love to Mom' and huge smiles of 'Good luck!' following me to the car.

Knowing my propensity for weariness on the motorway and worried that I was undertaking the journey solo, Her Most Wonderfulness had stocked up with essential driving provisions: cherry Coke and several bags of Fruit Pastilles. Having worked through lunch and into the afternoon dealing with the pastoral issues of a group of angry boys, I also had my uneaten sandwiches with me. By the time I had filled up at the corner garage before heading out on the A41 past the Baggies ground, I had added a couple of impulse-buy Double Deckers to my Motorway Survival Stash. With any luck, I might not have any need of them, but I was heading North, where everyone knows the weather can be perishing. I justified my calorific car load by telling myself that it might snow without warning, and it was better to be safe than sorry and musing to myself whether they had St. Bernard dogs, equipped with barrels of brandy, on the Yorkshire Moors ready to send to the assistance of snow bound drivers.

I was right to worry.

I stopped on the M42 for a comfort break, forgotten in my haste to get on the road, and added a huge hot chocolate to my supplies. No sooner had I rejoined the motorway, there it was, just after the service station exit: stand still traffic! I had not even reached the A42, much less the M1 that I had been dreading. I slurped grumpily on my hot chocolate, managing to scald my tongue, thus setting the tone for the entire journey. I was trying to reach Moosh and here I was stuck in a *grande bouchon*. Darkly muttering 'Shitty Death!' to myself and repeatedly testing my injured tongue, I inched northwards at a pace so slow that it would have embarrassed the laziest sloth.

Worse was to follow. Just short of Sheffield, the sluggish pace petered to a complete standstill. And there it stayed. I was over two and a half hours into a journey that I had hoped would take three, and I was marooned. Exhaustion from my early morning wake up overtook me, and I fell fast asleep in the middle lane of the northbound junction of the M1. When I lurched awake, mortified, the Bon Jovi CD had finished and restarted, and we were all exactly where we had been when I nodded off: standing still.

I have no idea what actually caused the bottleneck but, ever since that day, I have glowered darkly as Meadowhall Shopping Centre comes into view. I have had to strictly train myself to suppress the involuntary anger that mounts as soon as we pass Nottingham, because Sheffield comes next and, in my mind: Sheffield = Traffic Jams = Not Getting To Moosh.

When I eventually reached Loftus, dark had long since fallen and I had been on the road for five and a half hours. I was seething, mainly from the driving fatigue, but partly because I had hoped to pick up flowers near to Aly's so that they would be fresh for Moosh. Consoling myself by reminding myself that Moosh actually disliked cut flowers, associating them with death in general, but specifically that of her own mother, I passed Aly's and bought the biggest box of dark chocolate that I could find at the small supermarket. The thought of the gleam on Moosh's face when she saw the box managed to restore some of my equilibrium, before I turned back into Aly's driveway.

Out of all of the "real" houses that I have ever visited (i.e. owned by someone that we know as opposed to a house on *Escape To The Country* or, more recently, *A Place In The Sun*), Aly and Neil's house is my absolute favourite.

Woodlands is an imposing structure set in the middle of Loftus. Cavernous, capacious, huge, even humungous, it is *BIG*. Not as in stately home-sized, but a veritable warren of rooms radiating from a hall which can, on its own, comfortably accommodate a fair-sized house party and from which rises a glorious staircase purportedly designed by Charles Rennie Mackintosh. Downstairs, as well as a large kitchen, walk in larder, dining room that is home to a truly beautiful oak table, and sitting room, there is also a family bathroom, three reception rooms, a sizeable room set aside for Aly's provision of autism therapies and the Dogs' Room. Yes: *Dogs' Room*.

Walking into that party-sized hallway always makes me smile. It delights me that Aly and Neil managed to buy that wonderful pile, and its central hall symbolises Woodlands' potential grandeur. That evening, my smile was broadened by Aly's characteristic effing and blinding about the state of Yorkshire's motorways and the relieved and emphatic welcome she hurled at me as she emerged from the direction of the kitchen.

Simultaneously, hearing Moosh's excited squawks from behind me, thoughts of Sheffield began to be erased.

"Come on, she's dying to see you!" bustled Aly, urging me to put down my bags and ushering me into the reception room to the left of the vestibule (often home to at least one rabbit) and the unused but magnificent front door.

I was staggered and delighted by what I saw.

Moosh was perky and positively bouncing. She looked better than I had ever dared hope to see her again. Even without the predicted pleasure at the gift of dark chocolate, she looked sprightly and hale, and both Aly and I had to discourage her from lunging too enthusiastically, up out of her chair.

But that was not the prime source of my delight.

Moosh's room was wonderful!

Aly and Neil had created a home for her. Admittedly, of necessity, a much smaller space than her three-bed terrace in Shakespeare Road, but homely and full of Moosh's personality, very much *Chez Geraldine*.

Several of Moosh's most prized pieces of furniture were arranged artfully around the room: her father-in-law's beloved grandfather clock; the occasional tables that had been the focus of Granny Lanyon roundly chastising Aly and I, when we had proudly polished it with thick, purple floor polish; and her chaise longue adorned in elaborate period fabric.

In my entire life, I have never once thought to myself, "What we really need is a chaise longue. Doesn't everyone need a chaise?"

To me they are a pointless item, however, Moosh had bought it years before in Shrewsbury, as a consolation, retail gift to herself when she was infuriated with Dad about something. She was probably right to be cross, and ever since it had taken pride of place in her living room, so it was a must have in her new home.

Moosh's clothes were neatly tidied away but accessible to her, so that she could choose what to wear, thoughtfully giving her independence.

There was even Dad's beloved, antique, bedside commode in its lustrous walnut box. For years it had stood, pristine, lid lifted, in successive dining rooms, usually sporting a lush avocado or young orange tree, grown from seed by Moosh to stand in the ceramic bowl. Now it was ready to be used for its designed purpose: Moosh's nighttime wees.

Utterly entertained, I chuckled, "Does it actually work?"

Moosh's delighted grin was all the answer I needed.

Every available surface was covered with ornaments: displays of photographs of Dad, us and of course her grandchildren; silver tea service pieces; Granny Lanyon's tasteful collection of red glass evoking more memories of our childhood; and more. Those surfaces that did not hold ornaments were taken mainly by house plants. No longer able to tend her garden, I knew that Moosh would lavish care on the plants brought from her home, giving her purpose. Aly had even retrieved the Swedish Ivy that Moosh had been repotting on the night she made the newspaper bed in her kitchen.

Undoubtedly, the absolute *piece de resistance* warbled gaily in a cage facing Moosh's bed. A bright yellow canary sang its little heart out, its head cocked to one side, as if searching for Moosh's approval with its intelligent, black eyes.

"Another Jimmy?" I asked.

Ever since we were little, the homes that Moosh created for us always had at least one pet. She maintained enviably successful tropical aquaria in several of our homes. There had been a procession of dogs and later, when she admitted that dogs were too strong for her, Siamese cats. There had also been birds: several pairs of Australian zebra finches, always called Fred and Nina, and years and years of canaries, always called Jimmy, something to do with Dad's time serving in the Royal Signals.

"It wouldn't be a home for Moosh without a Jimbo, would it?" Aly beamed and so did Moosh.

I returned their grins, the tedium of the journey now fully forgotten and replaced with delight, "Isn't this brilliant, Ma?"

Clearly warmed by my response, Aly said, "I'm going to nip out for a ciggie, so that the two of you can catch up."

Moosh was not remotely shy about delving into the opened box of Black Magic I proffered and, mouth blissfully wrapped around a chocolate cherry confection, she looked deliriously content as I asked, "So how are you feeling, Ma?"

"Grateful," Moosh cooed around the mouthful. "I'm truly grateful. Alyson and Neil have made me very welcome and made my room lovely. They spend a lot of time with me, and Liam and Harvey do as well. Liam is very helpful too. He's been teaching me to use my wheelchair, but I'm still not very good at it. After hospital, it is so nice to feel at home, and I'm getting used to it not being my own home, the one that your Dad bought me."

As I formulated my answer, part of my mind was assessing and was reassured by Moosh's engagement and ability to articulate her thoughts.

"Aly very much wants you to feel at home and what they've done to your room is beyond anything I'd imagined, so it's good to allow yourself to feel that this is your home. Aly wants you here forever and is very keen to make this work for all of you. Are you behaving?"

Without missing a beat, Moosh said, "I have been very good. I promised you that I would be good, and I have been. You can ask Alyson."

We chatted back and forth, me sharing mundane updates from home and Moosh impressing me with her grasp of current affairs and the fact that she was back to being able to argue her Tory-leaning, political views. We were still nattering when Aly called through to let us know that she had ordered a Chinese and had asked for Singapore noodles for Moosh, who grinned on hearing 'extra spicy'.

Later, when we had settled Moosh for the night, Aly and I shared a bottle of heavy, fruity red wine, outside in the crisp night air and I asked, "Is it OK to say that I am dead proud of you? You have created a lovely space for Moosh. She says that she is behaving herself. Is she telling me the truth?"

Aly glowed in the dim light, "She has her moments Al. She can be a bit of an obstinate bugger. But, on balance, we are winning so far. It's early days, but we're winning. It feels right."

When I returned home, early the next afternoon, after a much better drive, I reported to Her Most Wonderfulness, "I think it is going to work. Aly and Neil have done an amazing job. Moosh seems to be settling and she appears to be trying to be cooperative. This might just work."

17

The Wheelchair

A fortnight later, committed to my promise of visiting at least every two or three weeks, I stocked up on calories and headed off to do battle with the M1, girding my loins for whatever the Sheffield stretch threw at me.

The journey lived down to my expectations; it was almost as torturous as my first Mission To Moosh. Having gained no benefit from setting out early on my previous trip, I left after school. The outcome was marginally better, but still nose to tail and exhaustingly slow. I cast loud expletives at Meadowhall, all lit up, as I tortoised past in the dark, wondering whether fellow voyagers could lip read my grim grumblings.

Once again, it was fully night when I arrived, late.

Once again, the reception was joyous.

Moosh appeared as vital as I dared hope. She was still a weakened woman approaching 80, who had clearly been through the mill in the last year, but she was full of smiles and chat and the mischief that was never far from the surface when she was on form. She reported that she was feeling more and more settled and was enjoying Harvey's frequent visits.

As if waiting for his cue or knowing that he was the subject of our conversation, Harv trundled into the room with his pen tapping on his fingers. He hadn't seen me arrive, so stopped in his tracks, before approaching for his customary close inspection of my features.

When he was satisfied that my hair met with his approval, I said, "Hello Harv."

"Hello Alistair," he replied, tapping.

"Hello Harvey," Moosh joined in.

"Hello Widget," Harv answered, turning his scrutiny to her hair. We all had our names for Moosh, but Harv must be the only person on Earth, who ever decided that it was appropriate to call his grandmother *Widget*.

Possibly wrong footed by my presence, Harv scooted off to find something else more entertaining than me, but Moosh told me that he came to check on her several times each day, systematically inspecting the position and orientation of each ornament on every surface and sitting down briefly on the edge of her bed or next to her chair. Moosh was certain that Harv was assuring himself that she was comfortable, and she enjoyed his proximity and attention.

Aly, too, was buoyed. For her there was enormous satisfaction that Moosh was taking to the environment that she and Neil had created. As we once again shared late night drinks outside, her smoking and us catching up, she fairly glowed with what was, in my book, a well justified sense of achievement.

114

"It is good having you here, Al. She needs you to come," Aly confided.

Pleased that Aly thought my trips were useful, I was disconcerted by an undercurrent to Aly's statement and turned to look at her, my expression inviting some elaboration.

"When you come, she lifts. She knows when you are coming and gets excited. You are The Golden Son, after all." There was no accusation in her voice, but a hint of fretfulness.

"She has ups and downs," she went on. "When you came last time, the up lasted a few days. Because she knew you were coming, the anticipation lifted her, but when she dips back, she is very weak, sometimes horribly weak. She gets terribly confused and disorientated, too."

Feeling a little punctured, I voiced one of my benchmark fears, "Does she know who you are?"

I knew, in myself, that I was dreading the day that Moosh could not recognise us. I was not sure how I would move forward, emotionally, if that point was reached. From previous conversations, I was very aware that Aly shared that angst.

"She does, Al. It's not that. It's more that she gets herself into situations that she can't get out of. Or, where she starts something and then loses the thread of what she was trying to do and finds herself terribly uncertain and quite afraid."

My sense of deflation magnified.

Now that she had started, and knowing that I was listening intently, Aly continued, "I think that she feels quite confined. Intellectually, she can rationalise that her frontiers have shrunk, but she is an intelligent person who, not so very long ago, was travelling the world, but now needs help to get to the bathroom, just a few metres from her bed.

"There are more and more times when even her hands won't do what she is mentally asking them to do. It must be horrific to be inside her brain not able to do the simple things. You should ask Liam about the wheelchair.

"Anyway, that's enough of me moaning. You don't need to hear my shit."

"I do," I insisted. "The least I can do is listen. You're the one carrying all of this, up here."

"It just gets hard, Al. It's hard to see her getting weaker. I don't mind her getting all excited about you coming, honestly I don't, but I know I have to be ready for the drop when you go home."

She raised her glass in a toast and leant against me, "It's good to have you here, Al, but it's scary shit! Here's to our little Mum."

Afterwards, I struggled to find sleep, due to interminable mulling over worst case scenarios. I was certain that it was beneficial for Moosh to be with people she loved and trusted, but worried that she would rapidly decline to a point when the emotional strain of looking after her would prove intolerable for Aly.

For both Aly and I, knowing that Moosh recognised us was of critical emotional importance. For myself, I could not see how I would continue in a caring role for Moosh, if she stopped knowing who I was. If that scenario occurred while Moosh lived with Aly, I would not expect her to do what I felt unable to.

After a fretful night, I was delighted to see Liam next morning. I needed his powers of making me laugh. As he had grown into being a teenager, his natural humour and storytelling prowess were fuelled by an ability to land himself in all manner of scrapes and precarious situations. He was a born mimic and raconteur, which rendered his recounts a joyous sharing.

I was still recovering from his recent telling of an incident in which he drunkenly found himself in a field surrounded by sheep. Uncertain of how he got there, but not wanting to pass up the potential for a comedic escapade, he first fixed upon the idea of sheep rustling. He has always harboured an inner Viking and, in his inebriated state, quite fancied the idea of roaming the Yorkshire hills with a sheep across his shoulders, or at least a lamb under his arm. Regrettably for drunk Liam, but luckily for the sheep, he quickly found that he was above the blood alcohol level that is detrimental to the effective rustling of a sheep (or even a lamb). Not hugely deterred, however, he decided that a spot of sheep worrying might be of some consolation. Just visualising his re-enacting of his disco-ordinated stumbling around a moonlit field of sheep, still makes me grin, but not as much as his trauma when the sheep took a fancy to him and decided that a bit of human worrying looked like fun and he had to find a way of getting out of the field without being able to sufficiently control his limbs to scale the walls. (N.B. Absolutely no sheep were harmed, although by the sounds of it, several were entertained.)

Knowing that there would be a tale to be heard, I said, "Liam, Aly told me to ask you about Moosh and the wheelchair."

His face cracked into a grin that was subtly tinged with something else, "Aw, Alistair, it was mint! Grandma wants

117

to be independent using her wheelchair, so that she can get around downstairs . . . you know, to go to see Mum, if she is in the kitchen, or, when she is feeling coordinated enough, to wheel herself to the bathroom to take herself to the loo without asking for anyone's help. It's good really that she wants to do things for herself."

Internally, I added Moosh's desires to continue to find ways to be independent to the already impressive inventory of positives that Aly had secured, by offering to look after her.

"She really wants to," Liam continued, "but she finds it hard. She was trying to shuffle herself along, using her feet to power herself and to get the wheels to roll around, while she is supported in the chair. Clever really. But she was rolling over her own feet. Not under the wheels but, as the chair moved forward, she wasn't lifting them and so her feet were getting stuck underneath her."

As he mimed it, making Moosh's scowlingly perplexed face, I burst out laughing, exactly as he intended, before he shamed me saying, "I know you shouldn't laugh –"

And then he was laughing too, "But it looked so funny, Al, and she was getting so vexed."

As we both hid our sadness, losing ourselves in the release of laughter, Liam persisted in driving his imaginary wheelchair and exaggerating his feet disappearing under the seat, before soberly continuing, "I said to her that it might be easier if she uses her hands to push the wheels. At first, she said that she didn't have the strength, but I sat in her chair and showed her where to put her hands and how I would push. She saw how easy I made it look and said that she'd give it a go, like. So, I put her in the chair and took her into the hall, where the wooden floor is smoother than her carpet."

Again, he grinned, but this time the sadness fully outweighed it, "Bingo! She was off. She fair shot across the hall and was all squealy with delight at her brilliance! But her steering was off, and she drove into the corner, when she was aiming for the door. It didn't help that I laughed, not realising that she was stuck. I tried to explain to her the mechanics of reversing, how to use her hands, but she could not fathom it."

More acting out of Moosh's face and unsuccessful reversing movements had the two of us chuckling, despite ourselves.

"Fair play though, she's a game old bird," Liam concluded. "She would not stop trying. Not then and not afterwards. The problem is, she still can't do it. I keep finding her stuck in corners that she has wheeled herself into. She's there, facing the wall, grizzling and, if I laugh, which I do, she calls me for being a disrespectful grandson."

I never did see her stuck in a corner, but I can imagine it. If I was there, I know that I would have laughed as well. Just like Liam, I find it useful to be able to find the funny in the sad. We were both more bereft than either of us would admit that day at the thought of Moosh so valiantly striving to retain her independence by mastering machinery that was new to her, yet failing. Both of us took delight in the fact that she still persevered, however vainly.

She was, as Liam said, a game old bird.

It was a good visit.

Moosh was much more up than down. Liam kept me

laughing and I was pleased that, however fleetingly, I was easing a little of the burden from Aly and that she enjoyed having her brother alongside her, knowing that I admired her effort.

However, as I once again drove away from where the hard work was being done, I worried.

18

Dinner In Loftus

In early December, Ranjit joined me for my M1 gambit to see Moosh.

We had decided to head up and back in one day, armed with sweets and fizzy drinks to keep me awake. As always, there was the offer of a bed for the night and a longer visit, but we wouldn't stay.

There are two reasons for us not accepting Aly's repeated entreaties to stay over.

Reason One is the Dogs' Room, or more fairly the fact that Aly is a rabidly fanatical Dog Person. Her Most Wonderfulness is, very much, not. When you put a doggy person, like Aly, in a house the size of Woodlands, there is the likelihood that the doggy person will fill the house with dog, either many smaller dogs, like a queenly herd of corgis, or one very imposing hound. Enter Milly, the largest New Foundland ever to have bestrode the Earth. Large, hairy and drooling adoringly at the sight of Aly, or of food, or at the very thought of food, Milly was never going to be loved by

HMW – she was almost the same size as Ranjit, a woman not brought up around dogs, a woman who just does not do drool.

(As a footnote to illustrate Aly's Doggy Person credentials: years later, when Milly had gone to laze in Doggy Heaven, Aly filled Woodlands with not one but three basset hounds! Just as drooly, but more like short, stocky, self-propelled battering rams, all floppy ears and lugubrious eyes, whose brains are clearly not connected to their direction of travel. Her Most Wonderfulness points to the proof of this, with abject distaste, citing the time that our eighteen-month-old granddaughter was mown down by a marauding Larry Dog, the last of the trio. Moo lay on the floor, startled and wailing, with a foot-long rope of drool looped over the top of her bare head.)

Reason Two, is even more basic. Woodlands is majestically cold. All of that ageing beauty requires a money pit that Aly and Neil just do not possess. Upstairs, there was more than enough space for us to stay in, with its laundry room, enormous bathroom and five bedrooms, so many bedrooms that one of them was actually a vast clothes room, before I had ever heard of 'walk-in wardrobes'. Heaps of space, but there were also single glazed windows. Single glazed windows in the north of Yorkshire equals frigid/frosty/free zing - take your pick. Her Most Wonderfulness is a woman who needs to be warm. She keeps her leg hair long beneath her leggings in winter, so that she can crochet it into a natural thermal base layer. When she is in bed, she needs to be hot enough to baste in her own sweat.

Much as we would want to take Aly up on her invitation, the combination of dog + cold + HMW dictated, "No!"

Consequently, I was very vocally, vehemently hating the idea of driving 400 miles in a day. Had we been driving in a southerly direction towards Mediterranean sunshine, I would have happily driven 600-800 miles, but we were heading north and so I was loudly bemoaning the likelihood of more traffic jams and hours of wasted life, but it had to be done. I consoled myself that the promised light at the end of the anticipated gloom of the tunnel was a tasty one: Aly was cooking us dinner.

On the radio, as we drove up the A42, there was a lot of excited noise about a Sheffield band, Arctic Monkeys, who had exploded onto the music scene. Having revolutionised the securing of their fan base through devotees sharing their songs and gigs on the internet, they had been achieving impressive record sales over the last year. As the worried parents of a teenage musician, we listened avidly. Alex had determinedly asserted that he would make his living as a musician; there would be no Plan B. As teachers with zero knowledge of the music business, we were always interested in how unknown musicians came into the public eye and found success.

Internally, for the sole reason that I now knew that it was home to promising musicians, I promised to look more favourably on Sheffield, once we reached there. In just over a month of upping and downing the M1, the Steel City had become confirmed as the embodiment of my hatred of the journey up to Loftus, as if that section of motorway past Meadowhall, prone to solid snakes of snarled up traffic, was in some way to blame for Moosh's ill health. Now I knew that it was home to this thrusting, exciting, relatively new band, maybe I could hate it a little less.

Despite merging smoothly from the A42 into the unexpect-edly unsnarled flow of traffic heading north on the M1 near Nottingham, I was muttering darkly to Ranjit that the traffic jams would be starting shortly, my mood not helped by Her Most Wonderfulness having adopted her bored-passenger pastime of radio station jumping. She had settled on a debate in which schools were, as ever, being identified as the place where another of society's ills should be addressed.

"You watch: there'll be no money. We'll be told it's already in our budgets. Bastards!" I growled.

My sense that something about the day was awry began as we traversed the Don Valley with no traffic disruption, and was confirmed as we positively sailed past Meadowhall. I swear the sun was gleaming on its green rooves, lending them a look of resplendent, aged copper, causing me to ponder that I had never seen Sheffield look so welcoming.

We turned into the drive at Woodlands in my PB time since Moosh's move north. Maybe I could hope that at least some future journeys would be jam free.

I almost skipped into the cavernous house in search of our hostess and keen to give Moosh a hug. My good humour rising even further as we neared the kitchen, drawn onward by a waft of roasting lamb.

Aly is an epic cook. She has never written a recipe book, nor been a TV chef or even tried out for Master Chef, but she loves to cook for a table full of people and does it in style, with verve and panache. Having had a catch-up natter with Moosh, I settled into the kitchen, helping out with prepping veg for Aly, and engaging in football chat with Neil, primarily the prospects of Reading, Villa and 'Boro.

Ranjit and Neil reengaged in their favourite activity, poking fun at each other, with HMW resorting to one of her stock mealtime digs by teasing Neil about when he and Aly first set up home together: she a fabulous cook and he a vegetable abhorring vegetarian, living on a trump-inducing diet of baked beans and cheese.

As potatoes were given their final, crunchy, gold crusting and the piping hot lamb rested, the juices being simmered and stirred into gravy, I was delegated to collect Moosh from her boudoir.

I bumped into Harvey, who was in mid visit and told him, "It's dinner time, Harv."

"Thank you, Alistair," he intoned, before leaning in for his full formal greeting: inspecting my features in minute detail, sniffing me and rearranging my hair.

Turning to Moosh, with a sense of all being well, I asked, "Ready? Teeth in?"

To which she pointed to her grinning mouth, displaying her dentures.

Then in a reversal of roles back to our childhood I threw in, "Toilet. Wash hands."

She chuckled, "That reminds me of your father."

"I know," I smiled. "Those Sunday dinners, with him cursing the beef. I was always glad to hear *'Toilet. Wash hands,'* because it meant that his swearing at the meat was over."

Now cackling, Moosh answered, "Just wash hands, please."

So, I trundled her down the corridor. I was still not entirely comfortable being in the bathroom with my own mother,

125

but the good spirits of the day allowed me to run the tap for her to wash her hands with minimal angst, knowing that I had got away without having to take her to the loo.

We all gathered, joined by Jess, which gave rise to more football chat, she being a truly ardent acolyte of 'Boro. There was a sense of almost pre-Christmas gaiety round the beautiful, sturdy table, which could almost be heard creaking, so laden was it with dish after dish of potatoes, vegetables, Yorkshires, lamb and gravy.

I sat next to Moosh, who was deferentially served first, and offered to cut her meat for her, knowing that her dexterity was no longer up to the task. She acquiesced, while I internally reflected, sagely, that maybe this was why hospital food on the geriatric ward was either sloppy or served in bite-sized chunks: the patients, not only being challenged in their chewing, but also having lost the ability to manipulate a knife and fork.

My task completed, I happily accepted my heart-endangeringly heaped plate, while Moosh set to, daintily spearing morsels from her plate and successfully manoeuvring them to her denture bedecked mouth. As I relished Aly's cooking, I watched as unobtrusively as possible, monitoring how Moosh fared and was pleased to see that she maintained a steady rhythm of fork to mouth, chew, repeat.

"Fabulous, as always!" I declared to Aly, although I was still faced with a small mountain on my plate.

"Delicious!" Moosh agreed.

So immersed in the positive trend of the day was I that I fully expected Aly to be aglow with pleasure. Consequently,

I was taken aback to see her accept our praise with a tight smile and a hardening of the eyes.

While the rest of us kept up a stream of further sharing of news and Liam's mixture of witty anecdotes and joking barbs at Neil's expense, Moosh ate and Aly was almost entirely silent, only answering if a comment was made directly to her. I tried to pull her in, but she remained distant.

The sense of something about the day being awry, rushed back: it wasn't the unexpected kindness of the M1 past Sheffield; something else was out of kilter, but I could not place my finger on it.

At the first opportunity to stand up and tidy away the dishes, I offered to help Aly.

Both carrying a weighty stack, I followed her into the kitchen. Even before she deposited her burden with a worrying crash on the work surface, I knew that she was crying. She remained facing the dishes, both hands gripping the counter, head bowed.

Feeling non-plussed, I tried to flank her, to be able to spy at least a portion of her face. It wasn't a good look, with clenched chin, pouting lips, inflamed eyes and a drip of snot threatening to fall from the end of her nose into the leftovers. I tried to turn her shoulders towards me, but she resisted, tensing.

Then she muttered, almost soundless, but there was no hiding the invective, "Bitch! Bitch! The fucking bitch!"

"Christ, Aly, what is wrong?" I asked, startled: I had been having a lovely time and, although I had sensed Aly's unhappiness, I was stunned.

Again, I tried to turn her, "Come on. What is wrong?"

127

But, again, I was rebuffed, angrily this time.

"The Golden Son returns!" Aly snapped, her voice still barely a whisper, but her ire abundantly clear. "Here you come. You cut her food. She eats it. What the fuck is that about?"

"I thought I was helping, Aly," I countered, unable to hide the defensive tone and a slight hurt from my voice.

"Yes! And then you'll piss off home and it will be me cutting her food and her refusing to eat."

She spat the words at me, furiously.

"I'll plead and she will still refuse. She'll play dead until I have to feed her and she'll still make it difficult. I almost have to do choo choo trains, as if she's a kid. And then you come and sit next to her, the Golden Son, and she fucking eats!"

Hurt welled up from her and I was her unwitting target.

"But she can eat!" I tried not to respond angrily. "You saw her. She ate. She ate well."

"I know! For you!" still spitting, but flagging wearily.

"For me, every mouthful is a battle, as if she is on hunger strike and I am forcing her against her will. You have no idea what it is like, Al, no idea!"

"That's true," I conceded. "I just did what I thought was necessary. Would you like me to talk to her?"

Aly gave the slightest nod, "Please. I don't know what good it will do, but would you?"

Heading back into the dining room, the mood was notably subdued, the conversation more muted. I looked to where Moosh and Ranjit had been sitting, and everyone except Harv pointed down the corridor. Ranjit had wheeled Moosh back to her room.

When I entered, Ranjit looked at me questioningly, while Moosh was a mixture of wide-eyed innocence and knowing guilt. I ushered Ranjit out with a subtle, sideward nod of my head.

Once she had left the room, Moosh looked up, saying, "It's me, isn't it? What have I done?"

"Don't you know, Ma?" I asked, almost imploring, wanting to avoid a battle. "Do you have no idea?"

"Dinner was nice. I ate it all, didn't I?" she answered. "I didn't make a fuss. So that can't be it."

"Ma? That's exactly it!"

It was a lot like talking to a child at school, who knew they were in the wrong and cornered and arguing their innocence.

"You ate without help."

"But you cut everything up for me," Moosh protested sheepishly.

"And you ate without help," I insisted. "Aly says that you refuse to eat without help. That you need her to feed you every mouthful and that, even then, you refuse to eat. You act as if you can't eat."

She drooped, "I can eat, but I like her to feed me. It makes me feel looked after. The longer I take to eat, the longer she stays with me. I like having her with me. I feel . . . loved."

"Ma! Aly loves you! We all love you!" I said. "You don't have to play games to make her love you. If you make mealtimes a battle, it will only make things sour."

Then, remembering her tactics as a grandparent, I tried to lighten the mood by adding, "It is not as if she can hide your food down behind the radiator, like you did for Arun and Ayesha when you were campaigning to be The Most Loved

Grandma In The Universe, is it? She has to make sure that you actually eat your food."

She laughed at that. We both did.

"I'll behave," she said. "I promise, Alistair. I'll feed myself and eat properly. Will you tell Alyson, please."

"I will, Ma, but I really think that you should tell her yourself," I suggested.

I returned to Aly, where she was noisily dealing with the aftermath of a feast for eight, banging and slopping tensely in a self-imposed total exclusion zone that silently forbad others to enter. I reported back Moosh's acceptance of culpability and her assertion that she would behave.

Aly snorted at that, but conceded a, "Thanks, Al, for talking to her. I'm sorry, but she just grinds my gears, sometimes. It is not always like this, but it's as if she knows which buttons to push and she looks like she enjoys pushing them and watching for the repercussions."

"Look, we are having her for Christmas, aren't we?" I said, trying to prod her onto a positive tangent. "Hopefully, that will give you a bit of a break. I will get here as early as possible, unless you want to meet me halfway. And we are having Moosh for the week. If you can get that far in one piece, we can try to give you a bit of respite."

Despite Aly accepting that this was to be looked forward to, the pre-meal levity was long gone, not to return. The non-understood portents of Sheffield's uncharacteristic congeniality had clearly been signalling the day's offness: we had all been looking forward to seeing each other, Aly had put in a mammoth effort, but Moosh had unwittingly scuppered the festivities.

Moosh's neediness was creating or re-exposing fault lines.

Jess had departed and the Woodlands males were, wisely, scarce, so Ranjit and I hugged Aly and Moosh and beat a hasty retreat southward.

As I drove, Ranjit sided with Aly saying that she, too, would have been gutted by Moosh's 'I want to be loved' tactics.

It was hard to disagree. And I couldn't even blame Sheffield.

19

Christmas

Christmas came in a blur.

I was not worried about Christmas at school. I never did. Our celebrations were always taken care of by others, not me. The Infant Nativity sparkled adoringly with gut bursting singing from our youngest children. End of term exhaustion did not decay into the narkiness or bitchiness that can sometimes happen when seventy knackered school workers are holding on for the holidays. The staff night out was characteristically raucous, but we avoided making our usual spectacle of ourselves. School was not a significant concern.

My brain was monopolised by four Moosh considerations: a) Could the dynamic between Aly and Moosh be oiled, so that life at Woodlands could run smoothly for all concerned? b) Could we create a Moosh space? c) What was the most effective way of getting Moosh to Birmingham for the holiday? and d) How would we get through Christmas?

I thanked goodness that the lack of school worries allowed me to focus on Mother Issues.

Even before the debacle of mealtime a few weeks earlier, Aly and Moosh and I had agreed that Moosh would spend her first Christmas away from her own home with Ranjit and me, back in Smethwick. We all hoped that this would give Aly and her family a bit of a breather, or, at the least, a week of respite, after having her live with them for two months. Although they had rapidly found ways to meet Moosh's needs, they were sorely in need of a break, some family time and an opportunity to regroup.

Aly reported that Moosh was keeping her word, as regards cooperating with eating.

"I think that she believes that you won't collect her for Christmas, if she doesn't at least attempt to feed herself!" Aly chuckled. "Call me a bitch, but I haven't told her that she's wrong. To be fair, she has appeared to be very contrite most of the time *and* apologised more than once every day. You should have been a priest, Al, just as she hoped, when we were young. She only listens to priests and you."

Aly's words were devoid of bitterness this time, but I was certain that the annoyance lurked not far beneath the surface of Aly's current equilibrium. I was relieved and encouraged that Aly was finding the resilience to be forgiving and affording space for Moosh to modify her demanding impulses, but my greatest fear was that Moosh's expectation of Aly, to be the dutiful daughter, would erode Aly's goodwill and undermine her sincere and heartfelt intention to provide Moosh with a home.

Aly had many positive attributes but '*dutiful* daughter' was not one of them, certainly not when measured against Moosh's early life experiences.

Moosh lived in Malaya until shortly after my birth, when she was 35: almost half her life. Although much of her life in Malaya was lived unwanted, away from both the bosom and the strictures of her immediate Hindu family, she had a plethora of painful experiences that shaped her perception of *daughterhood.* At the age of three, when her parents separated and pursued their respective new lives, she was placed in a convent, and she spent the remainder of her first two decades there, until recalled to her family to be part of, not her newly remarried father's household, but her paternal uncle's.

On the one hand, this afforded her the comparative freedom of working for the British army, but with it came duties, expectations and obligations. Under her uncle's roof, in the household where he was master, she acted as companion, maid and something unspoken. She enjoyed the fast car and handsome dog that were the rewards for the role, but there was a barely hinted at darkness to her brief, veiled recounting of those days. (I am deeply grateful that it was long after her death that I learned, from surviving female members of her Malayan family, of the darkly inappropriate expectations placed upon her - even six decades on, the women could only bring themselves to insinuate, obliquely, that these were sexual.)

She spoke in more detail, although still rarely, of the experience of young women she knew, who were described as the adoptive sisters of friends. To my perhaps naïve ears, I took adoption to be an entirely benevolent act, but Moosh's descriptions spoke of something akin to service. She told of young women brought into the home and given a roof, food and, if they were fortunate, friendship too. With these benefits came the roles of subservient playmate to the birth children of the family and additional maid for the household, frequently hard-pressed and often mistreated.

In her heart, the Moosh I knew was the feisty, Eurasian, ex-convent girl flying free, zipping around in her MG sports with her Alsatian, Fury, sitting in the passenger seat, both of their well-groomed manes being tugged by the wind. Sadly, somewhere else in her persona was a woman whose convent upbringing and intermittent contact with family had deeply embedded an expectation of the deference of the young to the old, of women to men and, critically, from a distance, of girls to their mothers. Staggering for a woman who, at the very most, had contact with her own mother for less than five years in her entire life.

I suspect that the die was cast young. Although what she witnessed in her early years of young women's roles within their families was very clearly distasteful to her, when presented with a daughter, and later still, a daughter-in-law, she reverted to the ingrained expectations of girls, and therefore daughters, that she had experienced before I was born: duty and service.

Having been abandoned as an infant and never having fully experienced her parents' families, Moosh craved love, but, apart from with Ayesha, where women were concerned, she found loving difficult and demonstrable love almost impossible.

Aly was, very simply, not like that.

She would never fit into that box, and she would resist any attempt to put her there. She wanted to help, even to serve, but entirely out of love and absolutely never out of duty. Her dream was that she and Moosh would become drinking buddies and confidantes and live out Moosh's last years as friends, an intergenerational, gloriously unhinged, *Hinge and Bracket*.

My hope was that I could ease the tensions created by Aly and Moosh's very different hopes and expectations. My visits were intended to alleviate the stresses, to take some of the burden from Aly, and to drop ameliorating thoughts into Moosh's ear. While there, I would help with Moosh's routines, take some of the load of paying Moosh the attention she craved, make a fuss of her and listen to any gripes.

Before the disaster of *the meal*, I had thought that this strategy was working, that I was giving enough support and nipping issues in the bud.

Part of my repertoire was taking Moosh out. Being an early riser, I would load Moosh into the car and take her off for a sunrise drive, either down to Saltburn or up over the hills and further to Whitby. Moosh had always liked a drive, but, after her perceived incarceration in Sheldon Block, these outings were true freedom. She commented on everything she saw, the stunning vistas, the farm animals, the trees that she would name as she had done with Alex, her lively interest giving me reassurance and hope.

The only dark cloud on those drives was Moosh's double edged gratitude, "Thank you for taking me out, Alistair. With Harvey, Alyson can't find the time."

"You're right, Ma. Aly has to think about Harvey too," I insisted, bud nipping. "Aly is doing so much for you, but to get Harvey into the car and your wheelchair and you, and to look after both of you would be impossible. You need to try to be reasonable, to try to understand. It can't all be about you. When I come, I can take you out, but you must not blame Aly for not being able to."

I guessed that there would be countless interventions like this to be made, if Aly's dream was to come to fruition. There would always need to be the oil of my diplomacy to alleviate the friction between the two of them. I promised myself that, if necessary, I would keep doing the same for years. I hoped that we would have those years.

By comparison, the logistics of decamping Moosh from Loftus to us was simple enough, despite my worries. Planning conversations between Aly and Her Most Wonderfulness resulted in an inventory of the various items that Moosh would need to be brought with her and a check list of actions that we would need to implement before her arrival.

At Woodlands, Aly took charge of gathering medication, denture glue and a huge box of pull-ups.

At our house, the tidy up was underway. Her Most Wonderfulness has a weakness for hoarding crap in any available space and had taken to storing oddities in our rear living room, items that did not yet have an identified purpose, but might one day come in handy. It was the same room that was already filled with surplus furniture, the children's X Boxes and Playstations and Alex's piano. I spent a couple of grumpy days, grumbling my way into each corner, making sense of the mess in order to create a space in which to move a stronger bed settee and make it possible for Moosh's wheelchair to navigate.

Looking at the room, once I had done my best, I had to concede that a) it was a far cry from the palatial splendour of the home in miniature that Aly and Neil had created for Moosh at Woodlands and b) the limited area of uncovered carpet that I had managed to reclaim from the joint detritus of HMW's stockpiling and the children's feral living was probably beyond Moosh's wheelchair driving proficiency. I would have to steer.

To minimise the driving commitment for both Neil and I, we agreed to meet at a service station, approximately equidistant, to exchange Christmas presents and a slightly drowsy Moosh. Once the Zafira was loaded with her, the gifts and enough Parkinson's related geriatric supplies to last a month, let alone the planned week, we made for home, worried about frailty, toileting and demanding behaviour.

Funnily, looking back to that week, after all the worry, what has lingered in our memories is Moosh receiving a stream of visitors, Midnight Mass, laughter and flying teeth.

Moosh was the centre of attention. Our friends, none of whom had seen Moosh for over two months and several of whom had not seen her for much longer, descended. Ranjit's sister, Narinder, and best friend, Teresa, our neighbours, Sally and David, and Moosh's friends from Church all made time to come to make Moosh feel special. She lapped it all up.

As my special treat to her and fearing that I might never be able to do it again, I swaddled Moosh in blankets and took her to the Oratory for Midnight Mass on her second night with us. I had worried that she would be too tired, but as soon as I suggested to her that I take her, she was vibrantly alive. We sat right at the front, near to the altar rail, and she beamed, even when she was lost in prayerfulness. It was a joy to behold.

Christmas dinner always involved Asti Spumante for Moosh. And Asti always made her giggle. The children were on great form and, when added to the Asti, had Moosh in fits of laughter. Arun and Alex kept up a dialogue of banter that would have given Liam a run for his money, and Ayesha dropped in her more subtle witticisms. They were naughty, really. Quite apart from taking great pleasure in seeing Moosh happy, they were making her laugh so that her dentures would fly out.

The first time it happened, Moosh was appalled, catching hold of her teeth just before they were completely out of her mouth, however her embarrassment was instantly overtaken by her storm of laughter as she wobbled them back into place. The rest of the meal and much of the rest of the week revolved around finding ways of triggering Moosh's projectile dentures and the tears of mirth that invariably followed. It was special.

Moosh was visibly fragile physically and she frequently dropped off into tired snoozes, but we were spared the worst of her frailty and had no fights over food.

But it was only a week.

For Aly, it was the rest of Moosh's life.

20

Babysitting Moosh

The plan that we formulated for after Christmas was that I would drive Moosh back up to Loftus at the end of December, stay overnight and return to Birmingham in time for New Year's Eve. Liam was playing a gig in Hull with Burning Rest, his thrash metal band, and I suggested that Aly & Neil go to watch the gig, offering to 'babysit' Harvey and Moosh; applying Aly's logic, how much more difficult could it be looking after Harvey alongside Moosh?

I had carefully quizzed Aly about what Harvey would need in the way of food and monitoring and bedtime.

  I was reassured that: a) he would not need any snacks, because he would have a proper meal before they headed Hullwards; b) he would happily play on his computer and read his books; c) although he didn't have an established bedtime, he would go to bed independently, when he was tired enough; d) I would only need to worry about Moosh; e) they would try not to wake me when they returned, so that I would be bright and breezy in the morning for the return journey down the M1, sneaking past Sheffield, before it spotted I was in the vicinity.

True to Aly's predictions, Harvey ate well with everyone else, before Aly, Neil, and Jess bundled off with Liam (in full dreadlocked, punk frontman persona) to set Hull ablaze.

Then Harv disappeared upstairs. After a few minutes I went to check on him and he was settled in his room, surrounded by a small sea of books and avidly watching something on his PC. I did not know how to fully engage him, so I gave him a quick thumbs up and went down to join Moosh to watch TV. She asked how Harvey was and I told her that he was settled and she said that he would probably pop down to see her soon. All was good and things were going swimmingly; I had this babysitting lark cracked.

Again, predictions came true. After half an hour, the door to Moosh's room opened and Harv came in, tapping his pen on his thumb.

"Hi Harv, are you OK?" I asked.

"Yes thank you, Alistair," Harv affirmed in his unique, endearing cadence.

"Hello Harvey. Are you having a nice time reading?" enquired Moosh.

"Yes thank you, Widget," came the reply.

"Are you going to bed? Can I have a hug?" asked Moosh.

Harv leant down, scrutinising Moosh acutely, moved her fringe to one side, kissed her ever so lightly on the lips and off he went.

"Will he just go to sleep by himself?" I asked. "Or will I need to do anything?"

Sensing my slight trepidation at the unknown, Moosh assured me, "He usually goes for a bit of a wander, until he is tired, and then he will go to sleep."

Babysitting Harv was only one of my responsibilities on that night; there was also Moosh to attend to.

After walking her round to the bathroom and leaving her until she called to tell me that she was done, I settled Moosh in, made sure that she had selected her tablets from the Quality Street box, checked that I was sure she had chosen all of the correct pills for night time, placed her book in easy reach and asked if there was anything else she needed.

She looked at me anxiously and tentatively requested, "Would you stick my teeth in?"

I waited for as long as I thought was reasonable for the Earth to open up and swallow me whole, but when I looked down at her, Moosh was still looking at me hopefully.

"You need a few blobs of the Polygrip," she advised shyly. "It's just there."

I hoped vainly that she was wrong and that there would be no box, or tube, or that the tube would be empty, but, alas, there was the box and there was the tube and it clearly held a goodly quantity of denture glue. There was no escape, so I gave in, picked up the box and accepted that I needed to read and understand the instructions, if I was to avoid gluing Moosh's jaw shut. With a sinking heart I read, quietly wishing that it was my eyes that were glued shut, then I reread.

"OK, you'd better give me your teeth, Ma. Do I take them out or do you give me them?"

"I can give you them," she replied, hands moving mouth-ward.

I turned away until she said, "Here, Alistair."

142

When I turned back, she had one little hand extended towards me holding her upper and lower dentures. Her other hand was held demurely over her mouth. My heart went out to her, seeing her embarrassment, which made me feel even more awful for being utterly repelled, as I cupped her teeth in my hands trying to ensure minimal contact with my flesh.

Feeling more than a little nauseous, I scuttled back to the bathroom and almost hurled the dentures the full four metres from the door to the sink. I then scrubbed vigorously with the toothbrush, telling myself that it was entirely natural to have foodstuff lodged between teeth, and challenging myself to look at my own teeth in the mirror, but knowing that I had licked them clean before I opened my mouth. I brushed harder, until I was certain that they were as gleamy as I could get them. Next, I dabbed them with a clean towel and then checked that I had left no whorls of towelling behind. Finally, I sat down on the loo and read the Polygrip instructions for a third time, looking closely at the helpful diagram and trying to calculate the size of the lines of glue in the picture, before giving it my best effort to replicate them.

Back in Moosh's room, I asked, "Shall I put them in for you or would you prefer to take care of it yourself?"

From behind her hand, still in place, she mumbled that she would do it, the embarrassment far from fading. Not wanting to increase her discomfort, I passed her the top set and, tamping down on my repulsion, forced myself to not turn away as she put them in place with blessedly little fuss. The lower set followed just as smoothly.

"Can you bite?" I asked, keen to know that I had done an adequate job.

She clamped her jaw shut, pressed hard and nodded.

"Do you want to test them on my hand?" I joked.

She shook her head, but grinned, stifling a laugh, her shyness thawing.

"My, what big teeth you have Grandma!" I exclaimed in my very best Red Riding Hood and her reserve fled as we collapsed in the release of laughter.

"All the better to eat you with!" she snarl-grinned with a flash of her teeth.

"That wasn't so very bad, was it? I didn't think I would be able to do it!" I admitted.

"I don't like asking," she admitted, too, with a gnarly-handed pat on my hand. "Thank you."

Our moment of denture-induced-love-in was interrupted by the sound of Harv running down the stairs.

I leapt up to check that he was okay, but Moosh stopped me saying, "He likes to have a run before bedtime. He goes up and down the stairs and has a bit of an explore. He's perfectly safe. He'll come and check on me again. You go to bed."

In the face of her calmness, I made my way up to my room, saying, "Night night, Harv," as he bounded past me on his way down, on one of what would be many laps of the house.

I settled down to read, checking on the clock after every page. Up and down.

I contemplated ringing Aly to check that Moosh was right. Up and down.

I decided to hold off breaking into their night of gigging. Up and down, up and down, up and down.

If I had tried to count, I would never have kept up. More

upping and downing.

Then there was silence, blissful silence. I held my breath, expecting this to be an interval, not the end, but no sound came. I exhaled and listened, trying to send my ears to every room in the house: nothing. Then I decided that, as the designated babysitter, I should check that Harv was in bed.

Stealthily, I opened my door and looked across the landing to his room.

The door was open.

Quietly, I walked across: no Harv.

I opened the door to Aly & Neil's room: no Harv.

He wasn't in the dressing room either, so I headed downstairs.

Moosh was awake, but hadn't seen Harv and reported that the last time he had visited was when I was there.

With growing trepidation, I checked the living room, the dining room, the room that Aly used for autism therapy sessions, the kitchen and even the larder which was mortice bolted against Harv's midnight food forays.

In desperation, I checked the storerooms and even went out into the yard: not a sight or sound.

I was failing in my duty.

I reported to Moosh that I could not find him, but forbad her from joining me in my search. The last thing I needed was for her to fall, again.

A voice in my head, now clutching at invisible straws, said, "Attic!"

Still no sound, so I headed up the stairs and had just made it to the door at the bottom of the attic stairs, when I heard a soft bump from the bathroom.

Hoping against hope, but mindful of scaring Harv, I just

managed to refrain from charging in, instead gently nudging the door open and there he was, in the solitary room that I had not visited, surrounded by a parade ground made up of every household cleaner you could ever imagine, and pouring a green liquid down the toilet.

The volume of my relief was only outweighed by the magnitude of my abject horror, which magnified severalfold as I tested the weight of the bottles closest to me: all empty.

Just then, I heard voices from downstairs. Aly, Nelly, Jess and Liam had returned and Moosh was filling them in on Harv's disappearance. I quickly assured them all that I had found him safe and well and took Aly to admire Harv's expert deployment of his troops, feeling slightly peeved at the speed of Moosh's reporting of Harv going missing.

It was 2:00am but, knowing that I was too traumatised to sleep, I decided to drive home.

Saying, "Goodbye and Happy New Year!" to the giggers and hugging Moosh, despite her minor betrayal, I promised that I would be back in a fortnight.

I always remember that night.

In one part of the world, it was the night that Saddam Hussain was executed. In North Yorkshire, you could find the cleanest, most sparkling, lemony fresh toilet that has ever existed, anywhere in the known world.

As I drove, I reflected that, between us, with Aly taking by far the greatest part of the strain, Moosh residing in Loftus looked feasible, immensely challenging but achievable.

Little did any of us know that Aly's phone call on the night of Ranjit's birthday party was less than seven days away.

IV

Part Four

Lightwoods Hill
February 2007

21

Transfer Deadline Day

As a head teacher, one of my most successful, winning characteristics had been naïve optimism.

For me, it worked both as a leadership strategy and a survival technique. I was forever signposting the way to ambitious success, endeavouring to convince my staff that, with their best efforts, we could achieve anything. Whenever the challenges of external expectations or poor data made things look grim, I continued to believe that, if we gave our all in our collective endeavour, the worst would not happen. Even when things did go pants, I believed that we could pull together to dig ourselves out of the holes that we sometimes found ourselves in.

So it had been on the Southbound carriageway of that motorway, heading away from my babysitting night. Faced with all of the stresses that Aly was under, I had not fully grasped how close we were to everything dismantling. I had not accurately read the signs. Either Aly had successfully obscured them or, in my optimism, I had not looked for them or, much more likely, had believed that I (in imaginary Superman pants) could support Aly to carry the strain and work around them.

From 200 miles away and visiting just once a fortnight, how could I have believed that? *Naïve*.

Following my January drive to the hospital at Brotton and then to meet with her and the social worker, Aly had been a true brick. Knowing that the pressure on her would soon be alleviated, she had been able to welcome Moosh back to Woodlands and, with the help of Lisa, a truly wonderful carer, had almost been able to enjoy the month up to the Saturday at the start of our half-term holiday, which had been identified as *Transfer Deadline Day*.

The key word being *almost*.

For years afterwards, it was too difficult to talk to Aly about her feelings in that month between her tearful phone call on the night of Ranjit's party and Moosh coming to live with us. It was an emotional 'No Go Area'. It was only after a dozen years had passed that I felt able to ask and Aly had the emotional capacity to share her conflicting emotions of anger, resentment, guilt and love - complicated love.

As Ranjit and I once again drove north, there were no thoughts about traffic jams or motorway misadventures: we were on a mission to bring Moosh to ours. We knew that we had planned to the nth degree for Moosh's arrival and decided to cross our fingers and hope that we had done enough. We reassured each other that there would be time to learn, to tweak and to make any major adaptations that were necessary.

Having listened to Aly's outpouring, even accepting that she was holding back much of the pain and had drawn a veil over some of the worst scenarios, we knew that, when we returned, our lives would be markedly, unquantifiably more complex. We had been a couple for almost twenty-five years, knew one another's strengths and believed that our relationship was strong enough to be exposed to what would doubtless be a major set of new challenges. *Naïvely optimistic*.

Nottingham, Sheffield and Leeds flew by without a negative thought. We made plans for a celebratory Chinese from Ki Ban to welcome Moosh to her new home, our home, and to mark the starting of a fresh, unblotted page for Moosh.

The only mishap of the journey to Loftus was when my trusty Zafira inexplicably slowed down, just south of Allerton Mauleverer, as if Her Most Wonderfulness had hurled a pair of invisible anchors out behind us. I nursed the car to the approaching junction, alternating between crooning encouragement and dire threats of scrapheaps in the sky. Hazard lights blinking, we trundled timorously up the slip road and pulled over, out of harm's way.

Never having been the most practical soul, as the engine idled, I guessed that I was in trouble and I had no clue what to do next. Having only ever called for roadside assistance on one occasion, I did not even know whether we were covered by the AA or RAC or someone else; anyone else. I fished through my wallet for a membership card, but found none. I switched the engine off and exerted a considerable amount of willpower to prevent myself from flapping and descending into gloomy mutterings about not arriving at Aly's in time.

Opting instead to light-heartedly laugh off my frustration, I quipped, "Maybe it's an omen!"

Her Most Wonderfulness then surprised me twice in seconds.

First, she laughed, "Positive thoughts only!" (Ordinarily, it would more often be she who mithered.)

Then she declared, "It has probably gone into Limp Home Mode. Try turning it on again."

"Are you making this up?" I asked suspiciously.

I thought it was only technophobe me who resorted to 'switch it off and switch it on again'.

"And what, pray tell, is Limp Home Mode?"

She was nearly right. I had never heard of limp mode, before, but it is a thing, and the Zafira had it, but I can't explain what it is. Doubtfully but willingly, I fired the ignition, surprised by the instant response. Amazed, I tentatively pulled back onto the road and then the motorway. I was expecting the same loss of acceleration, but the car was back to ramming speed and we once again raced north (observing the speed limit, obviously).

Not wanting to risk diminishing our optimistic mindset, I kept to myself my internal pondering about whether the car's hiccup was a portent of a doom, us stumbling from one problem to another. Or, was it a sign that, with Her Most Wonderfulness and me as a team, the gods would favour us and we would solve any problems with similar ease - *naïve optimism with bells and whistles!*

We pulled into the drive at Woodlands in good time, tooting the horn.

We had suffered no further mishap or car-induced interruption.

Before we climbed out of the car, HMW reached over, placed her hand on my arm and beamed, "Come on. Let's go get Geraldine and take her back to her new home."

My surge of gratitude caused such a lump in my throat that I was unable to speak, but I managed to mouth a silent, "Thank you."

The atmosphere inside the house was a subdued swirl of mixed emotions; Neil's practicality in identifying what had been made ready to be carried to the car; the relief that emanated from Aly in pulsing waves coupled with barely disguised anger, accented by her forlorn sense of failure and all of it bruised with regret. From Moosh there was the sullen resentment of rejection, ameliorated a little by her gratitude for Aly's attempt to give her a home. From HMW there was the purposeful bustle of toileting Moosh, ensuring that we were fully stocked with drinks and checking the small pile of items to be taken. Harv was unsettled by the activity and highly sensitised to the interplay of largely unspoken feelings. I simply wanted to leave, excited to be taking Moosh with us but, more pressingly, wanting Aly to have her house to herself and start to heal.

I fervently hoped that she could.

We were to take the essentials only: medication, pullups, clothes, a few favourite ornaments, the most treasured photographs, her wheelchair and Moosh.

As HMW and Neil attended to transporting these to the car and Liam wheeled Moosh out, not yet trusting her to steer around the corners in the corridor, Aly and I lingered in Moosh's room. Almost everything was remaining, including Jimmy, in the hope that, when time had passed and hurt subsided, I might bring Moosh to visit and maybe stay overnight.

Surveying Granny Lanyon's red glass pieces perched neatly on their table, Moosh's beloved chaise and Jimmy in his cage, I hugged Aly and sought to pierce her despondency, "You gave it a blindingly good go."

Once I had Moosh safely belted into the back seat and HMW was sat next to her, ready to keep her company and provide her with beakers of drink, Aly manoeuvred herself into the car doorway, the discomfort from her back etched large on her face.

She reached her arms around Moosh in an almost painful embrace and whispered, "I do love you, so much."

"I know. And I love you, too," Moosh answered. "I *am* sorry. Truly, I am."

22

The Descending Moon

Our preparations instantly reaped good dividends.

Moosh liked what we had done with her room, despite the comparative lack of space after her palatial lodgings at Aly's.

She approved of the positioning of the bed in relation to the TV and the window. She appreciated the fact that there were chairs for us and other visitors to sit in, so that she knew that she would not be in that room all by herself. More than anything, she loved the personal touches - photos of her and our Dad, of her parents and of her with her grandchildren; five crucifixes positioned above the door; her Oriental tea jars on top of a little wardrobe in one alcove; her shell collection, junonia and hundreds of tiny cowries in a square vase and much chunkier cowries, clams, sea urchins and her beloved tiger-striped nautilus in a basket; her dozens of stone and wooden eggs in a large bowl; her collection of dangling crystals in front of the French doors to catch the early morning sunlight; the pots of early flowering plants just through the French doors and lastly her missal and prayer books on an occasional table next to her wingback chair.

Moosh and I practised the toilet run, along the route that I had created by reorganising the kitchen, tucking the dinner table tight to the window and removing the plethora of items that HMW was prone to stashing in an ever-tumbling jumble just inside the door. Now there was a clear, safe, sufficiently wide route between the table and my Victorian school cupboard, claimed from my classroom when my last school was renovated, and now painted a fetching blue.

When I was a child, Moosh and I used to pretend to tango so, now, Moosh and I adopted a ballroom dance stance of me leading, walking backwards, with her hands on my shoulders and her feet following mine, out of her room, down four metres of corridor to the kitchen, past the blue cupboard on her right and the sink and cooker on her left to the narrow utility area where the bathroom was to her right.

The bathroom itself was going to be tricky, requiring me to remind Moosh to hold on tight, allowing me to release her with my right hand to open the door outwards, then go back into full hold to allow a 180° rotation, before reversing her backwards between the tiny sink in one corner and the truly gigantic steam shower unit, diagonally opposite, through to stand with the toilet behind her. Once the physical element of the endeavour was over, came the embarrassment of undressing my own mother.

A major factor in things becoming more difficult for Aly was that, since my last Loo Run on Sparkling Toilet Night, Moosh's condition had declined to the point of needing assistance with dressing and undressing, including when she needed the loo.

So here we were, son and mother, with me practising clothes removal – I could not allow the word 'stripping' to enter my head.

Ranjit and I had discussed who would take Moosh to the toilet. She had volunteered to do them all, for the sake of Moosh's modesty, but we had both agreed that I too would need to be able to do the Loo Run, because we recognised that there would come a time when Moosh would need the loo when Ranjit was not around to support her.

I looked down at Moosh with trepidation and she began to giggle, releasing me with one hand to make sure her teeth stayed in. I caught her weight, just as she began to swivel, and she giggled harder.

With precisely no help from an increasingly mirthsome mother, I righted her, held her up and pleaded, "You have to help me!"

"Yes Boss."

She couldn't stop laughing, but she did hold still, while I unfastened her trousers.

"If you do the trousers, I will do my pants."

What a relief. I would leave her to perform the delicate acts of knicker removal and replacement, which would preserve her dignity and stop me having to see her most intimate bits and pieces. I told myself that, when we got to the point that Moosh needed that level of support, Ranjit would be willing to do the necessary.

With her business done, Moosh and I retraced our steps without any mishap, despite her dissolving into more laughter as we danced back down the corridor with a couple of tango head flicks thrown in for good measure. By the time I got her to her room, she was good for nothing but chuckles and chortles and collapsed into her chair.

"Well, you were a big help, weren't you?" I berated jokingly, finally giving in to the infectiousness of Moosh's hilarity as tears rolled down her cheeks.

"But we did it!" she declared, with a triumphant nod.

As part of our Moosh-readiness, we had stocked up on Polygrip, which I was now expert at applying. We also had adult pull-ups, due to the onset of nighttime incontinence, and pots of Sudocreme for her bottom. There was Savlon and Moosh's favoured shampoo and soap, Pantene and Pears. It looked as if we were setting ourselves up in competition with Lloyds or Boots, with two shelves in her wardrobe neatly organised with sufficient of each product to outlast either of our high-street rivals.

Moosh's bottom needed Sudocreme to treat bed sores caused by sitting and lying. It was a source of further angst on my part. In my mind, Sudocreme is for babies' bottoms. I was always a very hands-on Dad, doing at least my fair share of nappy changes, so Sudocreme was a familiar ally in the battle against skin irritation, but now, deep inside, a growing part of me was quivering with dread. That quivering magnified every time I tried to push away the visions of Moosh on an adult-sized baby-changing mat with me sorting her out. There is world of difference between creaming your baby's silky bottom and dealing with a granny bottom.

In my world, bottoms can be a source of great hilarity. Our friend, Jayne, will attest to this with a pained gurn on her face, as not a year has passed in the last eighteen, without me warbling *Blue Moon Of Kentucky* to her at least once, in fond memory of the camping holiday on which she was all flustered by her ill children, who had caught a bug. She had rushed into her tent to grab a minute to get changed and unintentionally mooned at passers-by, having forgotten to draw the curtain. In my defence, I'm not the only one who reminds her of this; the memory has brought numerous moments of shared giggles to eight or ten of us for all of these years.

I've always been too shy to be a public mooner. I've never been one for sticking my bum against the coach window on the way back from Alton Towers or to waggle my buttocks at other users of the M5 heading to Glastonbury, although I do admit to the occasional, daring flaunt of my bot to HMW from the garden, if I'm certain the neighbours are not watching. She always cackles, before warning me in faux scandalised tones that police helicopters routinely hover over our garden to keep tabs on me.

Old lady bottoms are a whole different level of hilarity due to a single shared moment when I was about four years old. Granny Lanyon was visiting us in Cyprus and she was sharing a bedroom with Aly and myself. I have wracked my brain in vain to work out why both of us would have been relegated to sleeping on the floor, but nothing comes. What does come, vividly, is the memory of Aly and me, looking upwards, eyes wide, as a white night dress descended too slowly to hide Granny Lanyon's very wrinkly bottom being caught in a spot of light. If you Google "pickled brain", you will get a pretty decent impression of the image that was hovering above our astonished, young faces. Ours was an upbringing which placed more than average importance on modesty, so Granny mooning was beyond the bounds of naughty and we were lost in squeals of laughter. I think we were scolded for our rudeness, or silliness or just for being awake, but nothing could take away from the deliciousness of the forbidden mirth.

I share these 'bottoms are funny' anecdotes as a counterpoint to the wave of terror that afflicted me on Moosh's first night with us, when the Sudocreme moment was upon us. Somehow, I had swerved the need up to now, but there was no putting it off. HMW had reminded me of the necessity and then double-reminded for good measure. There was no way that Moosh and I were getting through the night without this pivotal moment of role reversal - a son tending to the derriere of the mother who had, no doubt, cooed at his own peachy tush decades before. The tub seemed to be growing and the label appeared to be luminescing a 'use me' message. A meaningful conversation was required.

Holding my embarrassment in check, I asked, "Ma, what do you think is the best way of me Sudocreming your bottom?"

I was certain that lack of agility would rule out Moosh lifting her legs up to her chest, like a parent holds their baby's, but the vision of potential exposure that image conjured up led me to swiftly suggest, "I was thinking that I could roll you onto your tum and put the cream on that way."

"That would work, but my tummy's been sore today," she replied. "Can you put it on, if I stand up?"

"Ma, you can't stand!" I blurted. "That's why you have a Zimmer and it's why I help you to move around."

"But I could use the Zimmer to support me," she suggested.

Frankly, I was willing to try anything to avoid the legs in the air option, so we agreed that I would undress Moosh down to her underwear, she would put on her nightie and remove her knickers, then I would help her to stand up, she would support herself by holding on to the Zimmer, and I would cream her derriere and help her to step into a pull-up, before hoisting them up for her. What could be simpler? What could go wrong? Minimal embarrassment.

It so nearly worked!

We got to the knickers-off, Zimmer support position, with me kneeling behind Moosh faced by her old lady bottom, her hands gripping the bar of the frame and my fingers generously daubed in Sudocreme. Without warning, I was transported back to that bedroom in Cyprus and was barely able to stifle a snort.

"What's wrong?" demanded Moosh.

"Nothing," I promised, beginning to liberally daub cream on her nether end.

I needed to crouch down to make sure that I was getting the cream into all of those folds and crevices that suddenly reminded me off a giant, white walnut. That damned snort returned and I failed to supress it. I attempted to turn it into a cough, but Moosh's embarrassment receptors kicked in.

"Are you laughing at me, Alistair?"

"No!" I promised with all the sincerity that the next snort allowed.

I had applied enough cream to ensure that we kept the manufacturers in business all by ourselves and it wasn't soaking in.

And then it happened!

At first, I thought I was mistaken, because the first movement was so gradual. Surely, Moosh's backside could not be moving towards me, downwards to where I was kneeling right back on my haunches. But, yes, it was coming my way;

a white, wrinkly moon was drifting down towards me! I gripped the only thing I could, Moosh's bum cheeks, and pushed back upwards to support her, desperately trying to lift myself against her small, but compact, weight.

She was caught between laughter and panicked wails of, "Catch me!"

The lashings of Sudocreme on my hands and on her descending moon made purchase difficult, but I managed to arrest her fall by perching her bottom on my shoulder, cocking my head into the small of her back, and putting my hands round her onto the bar of the frame.

"Gotcha!" I gasped with relief, positioning a pull-up on the floor and ordering, "Quick. Lift your right foot," positioning her foot through the leg hole. "Now the left."

With her still wedged between me and the Zimmer, I lifted the pull-up into place.

We promised each other that we would get better at this and hoped that Moosh's tum would be less sensitive tomorrow, allowing her to lie on her front.

Just before I left her, in a moment of belated genius, Moosh suggested that we could have tried lying her on her side and we both fell into further giggles as we berated ourselves that we hadn't thought of the lying-on-her-side option earlier.

23

John's Counsel

For several years in the 90s, my and Her Most Wonderfulness's Friday night routine had been to meet up, in a group of four couples, for beer and food and companionship. There would be work chat, political debate, mundane sharing, amiable banter, friendship and constant mutual encouragement.

Those Friday nights were a happy, anchoring fixture of our early parenthood years.

Jayne (of *Blue Moon Of Kentucky* fame) and John, were one of the four couples. Our relationship, as a pair of couples, was predicated from its first few interactions on banter and the ability to share deeply personal matters. It still is.

We had known Jayne from our college days and then, when I moved to my second school, I found that Jayne worked there and our friendship grew, as work colleagues and then car-share buddies, and being part of the long-lost teaching tradition of Friday lunchtime dashes to the nearest, passably decent pub to herald the end of the working week.

One Friday, with our group of lunchtime escapees huddled

around our usual tables, Jayne took us all by storm by announcing that she was going canoeing at the weekend. Our initial reaction was utter shock that our friend, who eschewed all forms of exercise other than a good bop, was going to venture onto a river, paddle in hand, and exert herself. Surprise quickly morphed into suspicion, as the gossip radar in the group nagged away at the 'why?': why was a devoted non-exerciser and disdainer of mud planning to put herself through a camping activity weekend with the odds-on certainty of a dunking?

It was quickly decided (*not by me*) that, for this sea change in behaviour to take place, a man must be involved! The confirmation of Jayne's blushes led to a raucous chorus of the *Hawaii Five-O* theme tune, accompanied by much comedy paddling in the small amount of space around our tables. We were still paddling vigorously as we wended our way back up the lane between the scrap metal yard and the school field.

The man was John, and, once we were introduced, the banter and laughter between us began almost instantly.

One of us invited the other to play golf at Warley Woods, the little golf course close to where we lived. I loved a recreational, after-school game of golf on summer Wednesday evenings. It must have been an invitation rather than a challenge, because I knew I was awful. However, I would have happily agreed, because I loved the leisurely pace and amiable camaraderie of meeting up with friends that golf afforded. Looking back to those less work-frenzied days, I still find it hard to believe that there was a golden period in teaching, when it was possible to go to the pub on a Friday lunchtime and take time, mid-week, to get to the golf course *before teatime* for nine holes, but we did.

I was most certainly not ready for golf with John. Even before we teed off, his warm-up routine of intimidating stretches and swings indicated that he had a far better idea about what he was doing than I did.

This was confirmed by the mighty swipe of his first tee shot with a long iron that launched his ball straight up the fairway (a route I wasn't used to) to become a distant speck in perfect position. I applauded, genially.

The camaraderie of our nascent friendship lasted all the way up to my second shot, an abortive hack. With my other golfing buddies this would have been met with polite commiserations. With John it brought forth undisguised hoots of unapologetic laughter.

And so it continued, with my sustained ineptitude affording John one opportunity after another to guffaw at the misfortunes that I brought on myself and keeping gleeful count of the trees that I struck on a very wooded golf course. In fairness, he was also well able to laugh at himself, being prone, despite being a far better golfer than I, to the occasional spectacular slice to the distant right.

Over the years, when he and I played, I almost always managed to bring John's golf down to my incompetent level, so that, although a much more proficient golfer, he only ever beat me by a small margin – maybe he was being kind. I have beaten him precisely once, a truly glorious, but lamentably brief event, culminating in me driving a ball an unfeasibly long way (for me) over a French lake. It is seared into my golfing memory, much as Paul McGinley must recall his Ryder Cup winning 10 footer at The Belfry: if I close my eyes now, I can still see that ball flying!

Our years of golf etiquette-breaking have provided us

with countless hours of fun, which have seen us shushed on courses from Derbyshire (my old school friend, Dominic, and I rolling around on the fairway after John's abortive chip attempt out of a green side bunker) to Brittany (John and Dominic calling *'le singe est dans l'arbre'*, to the amusement and bemusement of French golfers, at every shot that veered into the pines, so much so that golfers in that part of the world probably still cry 'the monkey is in the tree!').

Despite the hilarity, however, it has been the more personal conversations on those outings that I have cherished most.

Just as our Friday nights at the Wagon & Horses interwove banter with more serious personal exchanges, so too our golf games. Most of the conversations were light-hearted meanderings in much the same way as my golf shots would take us this way and that way across the course. Others were more serious sharings of life's challenges. On many golf evenings, we would sit next to the 7th tee waiting our turn, admiring the way the woods were lit by the setting sun, as we unpicked work issues, or discussed family matters.

I came to value John's advice and the fact that he was brave enough to engage in difficult conversations. He has a willingness to be there when he knows that times are difficult, and an unerring knack of visiting when needed.

Over the years, in amongst the laughter that has characterised most of our interactions, we have cried.

Not long after Moosh arrived, knowing that a review was scheduled and that it was a scenario that his job made him far more conversant with than I, he had rung to give me pointers for the meeting. As a result, I was well prepared for the review and found it supportive and constructive, however, some of the messaging from professionals about how Moosh's needs might develop and the challenges that we could expect had been bleak.

Without suggesting that he would, John broke his journey home to come to ours to find out how we were, after the review. He listened to me unload my concerns about supporting Moosh and my thoughts about what might be best for her, and outlining the decisions that we would have to make. He knew that I was struggling with the import of the meeting and the burden that the future appeared to hold.

Without shying away from my worry, he suggested, "Mark, we've reached a point in our lives where our roles around our parents have reversed and it is our turn to care for them. We will be called upon to make many difficult decisions. All we can hope is that, when we come to bury our parents, we can stand beside their graves and say that we did everything that we possibly could for them."

Many, many years before, on the day of the most scaldingly honest conversation we ever shared, my post-traumatically stressed Dad gave me the most impactful piece of advice I have ever received, when he entreated me, "Be a better father than me; spend time with your children and talk to them."

It is advice that shaped the parent I have sought to be.

So too, as Moosh's son, John's counsel would be at the root of my behaviour over the coming years. From the day of Dad's death, I had accepted that Moosh saw me as her protector. Now, I readied myself to be all that Moosh needed; I accepted that it would be hard, but I vowed that I would give it everything I had.

24

Carole's Verdict

Our school was a family. I know that many workplaces make that grand claim, but it is very often a top-down branding. At school, I was deeply proud of the fact that the description came from Sophia, one of our teachers.

Sophia was rarely visible for much of the year, just quietly beavering away in her classroom and then racing home to support her beloved father and her siblings. But once a year, for many years, she emerged, transformed into Cecil B. DeMille, to put on our Easter Service.

The first year that she took on this role, either I had asked her to, or she had offered to, as part of her Religious Education Coordinator responsibility. We had a brief conversation about what the service might look like and then I left her to it. The glimmer in her eye failed to warn me of what was in store. Think DeMille's biblical tour de force *The Ten Commandments*, boasting some of the most epic sets ever created for film; recall its cast of thousands, and you will be some way towards envisioning Sophia's directorial debut.

Traditionally, it was my role to stand up to introduce the assembly to our school of 420 children and our staff and many parents. Little did I realise that well over a third of the children actually had a part, from the Year 6 children who had bagged the starring acting roles all the way down to the 60 Reception pupils, who joyously waved palm leaves nearly as big as themselves. It was so DeMillesque that you could almost taste the sands of the Sinai desert, and, although it didn't quite have the same 220 minute running time, at an hour it was beyond the bladder control of some of the more exuberant palm wavers.

Although I fondly dubbed her *Cecil* for the remainder of our years of working together, and, each year, teasingly tried to prevent her from pulling passers-by from the street to bulk up the cast, the crowning glory of Sophia's Easter production was the prayer that she wrote to close out our Service. In it she sought to capture our wonderfully multi-ethnic school, which boasted every major world faith and many smaller ones and was home to approximately forty languages. She hit upon the line that would define us ever after: "Coming together as The Family Of St. James".

That phrase, *The Family Of St. James*, was quickly and affectionately coined by other staff and myself and was soon being used by the children in conversations and their writing about the school. Often, in future assemblies, when children used the phrase independently, staff would catch my eye and there would be a moment of pride in the sense of community that we were instilling.

One September, I received a letter from a Year 7 boy, who, in truth, had not always been the easiest youngster to manage.

Written in his very best and entirely unique hand, he spoke of how well he had settled into secondary school, but then expressed how he missed "the closeness of *The Family Of St. James*". Proud tears were shed in my office by members of staff who popped in over the following week, mingled with prouder smiles, when I shared his sentiments with them.

That lad was absolutely spot on: there was a closeness amongst *The Family*. This closeness was constantly demonstrated by the staff, many of whom shared deep work friendships, while others carried their friendships out of the bubble of school into their real lives. We shared our joys but, crucially, supported one another through the pressures of life, carrying those in need through challenges and losses: emotional traumas, health crises, marriage breakdowns and bereavements. Many was the time that people would arrive early or leave late for the express purpose of providing succour to a friend in need.

The lives of staff outside of school did, sometimes, intrude on work. Some argued that this could go too far: there were more than a few moments when one or other member of the team opined that another member needed to get back to focussing on the task at hand, work.

On one occasion, the difference between the way we did things and the way things were done in other schools was thrown into stark relief, when I was carrying out lesson observations with a colleague head teacher (judging the quality of teaching and learning in lessons) and stated that we would not disturb a particular lesson, because the teacher was in class teaching, but was struggling with a life situation and I did not want to add to their stress. We did not observe the lesson, but the comment was made by my colleague that she had no knowledge of the angsts that beset the lives of her staff, as they were not to do with school. My view was that, while valuable and expensive time was taken by tending to the life needs of members of staff, on balance the school benefited from those staff being given time and love to work through the challenges they were facing, because they would, when necessary, show a similar, or even greater, care of the children's and parents' needs and for those of their workmates.

We did know possibly more about one another's lives than is common in other workplaces or maybe just other schools, but, time and time again it was demonstrated to me that we were onto something life enhancing.

As Ranjit and I navigated Moosh's move, without expecting to, I became the beneficiary of care from my school family.

Even though I was 'The Boss', I was repeatedly reminded, "Mark, you always tell us that life and family must come first, now it is time for you to put your own family first."

In Moosh's time with Aly, when I was haring up and down the M1, doing battle with Sheffield, or meeting with social workers, the leadership team and admin team had picked up my responsibilities for me, ensuring that the school did not suffer. As we prepared for Moosh to come to us, I had not asked for my situation to be treated in confidence and so, as these things do, news spread. Soon, almost everyone knew about The Big Move and the support was heartfelt and heart-warming.

Pretty much every day, my passage around school brought enquires into Moosh's current state of health. Our front of house team, entirely of Asian heritage, would never let me pass without a 'How's Mom?' And I was jovially and lovingly berated as an unbefitting, pseudo-Indian son, if my light-hearted, deflecting response was in the realms of 'Mad as a bag of frogs!'

I carry that warmth with me to this day, some 13 years later, but the most vivid, fondly held, single example came from an entirely unexpected source: Carole.

Carole and I rubbed each other up the wrong way, often. We could be thorns in each other's sides and, much more than once, some very forthright views were shared in both directions. She was unashamedly, ardently, old school, revelling in her Victoriana persona, while she thought me a wet behind the ears newbie and a soft touch on children's behaviour.

When we would take children to The Black Country Museum as part of their History experience, Carole would say, "That was my life! That is exactly what Mother's house was like! That's what schools were like . . ." adding vehemently, "with proper discipline!"

Carole was the living embodiment of tough-love discipline. Her admonishment of misdemeanours was strident, but she always lauded her class as 'the best'. She loved the rogues in her class, because they knew which side their bread was buttered and were very rarely rogues for her.

Time and time again, returning past pupils would ask after her and tell me that she, too, was 'the best': "You always knew where you stood with Miss."

She was not the greatest fan of 'Management'(any manage-ment), seeing herself as one of the workers and letting me know that, as a manager, I had secured for myself a perch that she had no time for or truck with. She railed against anything that I did that she perceived as unnecessary interference in a job that she knew how to do, and was qualified to do, by virtue of her university degree. To make matters worse, she was a couple of decades my senior and so, while my upbringing taught me to be respectful and appropriately deferential towards her, she frequently let me know that she saw me as an upstart whippersnapper, who was trying to make a she-leopard change her spots and that 'just can't be done!' I adopted the strategy of never challenging her in public, but behind closed doors we had more ding dongs than I did with any other member of the team.

To be scrupulously fair to her, despite the shortcomings I had in her eyes, she could also be my very vocal advocate, announcing volubly in my hearing to any returning ex-staff, that I was, "The best boss we've had." (If only she didn't immediately diminish that by mischievously adding, almost with a pantomime slap of the thigh, "But that's not saying much, is it?")

What shone through with Carole, on the days that she riled me just as much as on the days that I admired her, were her strong values. She believed that all children must respect their elders and teachers, because of their position and because they were adults, whereas I believe that teachers must earn respect. She believed that the truth was the truth and should not be sugar-coated, even if it was difficult to swallow at first; I chose a path of diplomacy. We both believed that 'Manners maketh man', although we did not always agree about whether this had been demonstrated in the other's behaviour: me in questioning her snipes at colleagues or parents and she in her righteous wrath on the day her age dictated that a Retirement Workshop flyer be placed in her pigeonhole. The admin staff had been too afraid to be seen putting it there, so I took my life in my hands and did it myself, leading to indignant ire at what she perceived to be my ageist disrespect and loud assertions of, 'You want rid of me!' - sometimes her strong values worked in my favour, sometimes not so much.

And so it was one evening, as I was heading home.

About to drive out through the car park gate, I found myself obstructed by Carole. She was standing on the driveway talking with a colleague. Seeing me approaching and recognising that they were blocking my exit, I guessed that they would move, but Carole turned in my direction and held her ground.

Not knowing whether there had been any issues brewing and unprepared for a spat, I muttered portentously, "Oh bugger, what now?"

As she drew breath, I invisibly girded my loins, before lowering my window.

To my surprise she opened with, "I've said it before, Mark, and I'm not afraid to say it again: you're one of the good ones."

Inwardly, based on previous experience, I braced myself for the expected waiver, but she continued, "There's not many people as would do what you are. Nowadays the young ones discard the old as if they are inconvenient. You taking in your Mum is admirable. It is the way it should be, but too many people forget that. Good on you! I hope it goes well."

And with that, she stepped aside, silently indicating, "Now be on your way, young'un. Good lad."

In our school family, it was like being given an encouraging pat on the back by the recalcitrant matriarch, who everyone trod carefully around.

It did me the world of good, buoying me up for the weeks ahead, whatever they might hold.

25

The Morning Routine

Moosh had come to terms with the idea that some of her needs could be met by carers.

Her positive experience with Lisa at Aly's had gone a good way to overcoming her deep rooted resistance to outside interference in her life. She and I had spoken at length about how to use the allocation of hours that the assessment of her needs and our circumstances had afforded.

It was not only she who had reservations about her needs being met by carers. I felt strongly that, where possible, we should build Moosh into the family and that we would meet those needs that were within our capability. While I was reluctant for the children to be drawn into the role of joint care givers, Ranjit and I were determined to play our full part and only to take recourse to external support where necessary.

Together with the carers agency, we drew up a rota of visits to make sure that, once Ranjit and I were on our way to work, Moosh was given breakfast and dressed by carers, and that she was visited. Thus, meals, hydration, medication, hygiene and, crucially, company were all timetabled.

Moosh, as had been her life's pattern, was comfortable to be spending periods of time on her own. She acknowledged that she needed to modify some of her views and behaviours from her time in Loftus and that there was a need for others to help her to stay safe. In a moment of stark honesty, she volunteered that she had pushed the bounds of enjoying being looked after by Aly far into the area of taking advantage and being knowingly over-demanding - but insisted that she had simply been relishing feeling loved. She promised that I could tell her if she was slipping back into those behaviours.

The rota of carer hours did not stretch to every eventuality. I did not want it to. Being an early riser and knowing that Moosh woke early, I had timetabled myself for getting Moosh out of bed, making her a cuppa and administering her early morning medication, before heading off to work

It seemed that we had come up with a plan that had a good chance of success.

Those mornings, in that first month, were a simple, if qualified, joy.

I set my alarm to go off half an hour earlier and gave myself a serious talking to about speeding up my own morning routine of breakfast, wash, shave, shower, dress, by cutting out my half hour of staring vacantly at the TV over the rim of my cereal bowl – and it worked. Each morning, when I was already ready to go to work, I hung my suit jacket over the post at the bottom of the stairs and made tea, having set the kettle to boil on my way to get dressed. As I placed her beaker on the occasional table next to her wingback chair,

Moosh would already be rousing herself.

Being forty-five minutes behind me, Moosh's polite response would be rather more muted than my hearty, "Good morning!"

We both knew that there was one task that was required before we could properly enjoy a few minutes of quiet togetherness: the nappy change. It was not strictly a nappy change but, due to her incontinence not allowing her to get through the night without needing a wee, coupled with her not having the strength to be able to get to the bathroom unassisted, Moosh was now sporting pull-ups to prevent accidents in the night. Not wanting to suffer what she took to be the indignity of one of the carers finding her with a heavy pull-up, Moosh had asked me to change her out of the pull-up and into pants.

Being a veteran of the descending moon hilarity, I knew that I could inure myself to further visions of Moosh's behind, but it was never going to be the favourite part of the day for either of us.

Remaining in bed, Moosh submitted stoically to the nappy change. Each day I brought levity to the routine thanks to the electronic bed that the occupational therapist had arranged. It was a boon for Moosh and a fabulous toy for me. Using the bed's super responsive control buttons, I would raise her up and lower her down in quick succession, and then lift only her upper body and then just her legs: not quite how the controls were intended to be used, but great fun.

Clearly, this was not the most sensible move, because it would inevitably lead to loud protestations of, "You are a wicked man! You'll make me wee! What did I ever do to deserve a son as mean as you!"

She knew that her threats of weeing would stop me and make me focus on the task at hand, removing first her pyjama bottoms and then her pull-up. Each day, she attempted with varying degrees of success to help, by trying to raise her bottom from the bed. Pull-up removed, I would give her a quick wash and dry with a flannel and towel and she would roll onto her side to allow me to apply her morning lathering of Sudocreme. This still drew titters from both of us, and hums of *Blue Moon Of Kentucky* from me, but we were becoming accustomed to the task and much more grown up about our respective roles within it.

Finally, I would pop on fresh pants and her pyjama bottoms, rendering her ready for one of the carers to do the whole thing again later and dress her properly, without danger of them finding her in a wet pull-up.

Each day she thanked me for this task, and we chatted amiably before I took Ranjit her breakfast and her own cup of tea, and then set off for school.

That first month with us saw Moosh's incontinence worsening.

One morning, I came down to have my own breakfast, only to hear Moosh calling me from behind her door. It was not yet time for our morning routine. She sounded plaintive rather than in serious difficulty, but I rushed in flicking on the light, to find her trying to lower the bed, looking utterly abashed.

"I've wet myself," she whispered, clearly not wanting anyone else in the house to hear.

"That's OK, Ma. That's what the pull-ups are for, isn't it?"

"It hasn't worked. There was loads of wee!"

179

Her embarrassment caused her voice to rise to a barely supressed shriek, "I've soaked the bed! I'm so sorry!"

"Not to worry, Ma. Let me see what I need to do."

She was absolutely right. She was soaked. The sheets were soaked. Her pull-up was a lumpy, hefty weight. She looked appalled.

"Blimey, Ma, I think you've sprung a leak! We may need a plumber!" I tried to joke us away from Moosh's bereft expression. "I wouldn't believe that someone so small could have so much wee inside them!"

"Me neither!" she shuddered.

With an efficiency that gave me a flash of quiet pride, I folded a towel onto the seat of her chair, stripped Moosh of her wet garments, leaving them on the bed, wrapped her in her dressing gown and set her on the towel covered chair. Asking her to wait for me, I collected warm water and her flannel and another towel to give her an admirably efficient wash down. Next, I dressed her in a fresh set of underwear and pyjamas and resettled her in the chair, before gathering up all of the wet bedclothes and soiled towel and garments, together with the sodden pull-up and headed back to the kitchen, putting the kettle on to boil. Having set the washing machine going, I took Moosh her customary beaker of tea, a little early, and went off to get myself ready for school.

I returned to find Moosh sitting dejectedly, tea untouched.

Looking up at my arrival, she whispered, "Is this what I've come to? An old coot who wets the bed and has to be tended to by her son?"

I winced, not able to find a joke to make her laugh off her despair, offering instead, "Don't be too down on yourself,

Ma. We know there are going to be difficult times. We've broken through the barrier of going to the toilet and the Sudocreme and me washing you. I guess we will have to take each day as it comes. There may be lots of things that I have to learn and for us to get used to, but we've made a pretty good start."

"You're not disgusted by me?" she asked.

"Disgusted?" I shook my head vehemently. "Why would I be disgusted? It wasn't even messy. You're my Mum. I want to look after you."

"You promise?" she needed more.

I knelt on the floor next to her, "Ma, I'm not disgusted. I promise. But I do need to get going."

I touched her beaker, "Your tea is still drinkable. I'll see you tonight. I love you, Ma."

Heading to the door, I waved, before finishing, "If it's Florence, who comes today, can you ask her to make the bed? If she can't, I'll do it later."

When I came home that evening, the bed was neatly made and Moosh's melancholy had disappeared, replaced by an entirely more positive demeanour.

Before I had a chance to take my coat off, Moosh called me in excitedly, saying, "Look! Florence left those!"

Tucked tidily at the foot of the bed was a blue and white plastic wrapped bundle, much like a pack of toilet rolls.

"They are bed pads!" Moosh announced. "Florence assured me that big accidents do sometimes happen and it doesn't mean they will keep happening forever. She told me to say that, if we put one of these on my bed at nighttime as well as a pull-up on me, the pad will stop the bed from getting wet. She was very impressed, by the way, when I told her that it was you who sorted out my bed this morning. She put the wet laundry on the radiator. Is that OK?"

The transformation from the bereft mother that I had left to the reassured, encouraged one that now sat before me was such a relief that I wanted to ring Florence straight away, but I did not have her personal number. Instead I asked Moosh to tell her that she was our new guardian angel - she had always liked the idea of guarding angels.

That night we added bed pad placement to our nighttime routine and next morning we were delighted that, although the pull-up had overflowed, the pad was up to the task. Moosh took great pleasure in sharing its success with Florence.

Later in the week disaster struck again.

I came downstairs to find Moosh sodden. The pull-up was full, the bed pad had not been sufficient to catch the overflow. It looked as if Moosh must have inadvertently moved over to one side of the bed, so, once again, sheets, pyjamas and towels were put into wash and pull-up and bed pad were thrown in the bin.

I masked my frustration and, instead, calculated that, if I simply accepted that an incontinent Moosh needed more of my time and set my alarm another fifteen minutes earlier, we could navigate soggy mornings.

This time, however, far from being defeated, it was Moosh who suggested, "How about using more than one pad? That way, if I move, hopefully the extra bed pad will catch the wee."

Rather brilliantly, her suggestion, together with another

from Guardian Angel Florence, did the trick. Florence signposted me back to the occupational therapist who allocated a commode, which we placed next to Moosh's bed. Moosh invited all sorts of people to sit on her commode throne and howled in a most unbecoming fashion when I decorated its institutional plasticness with bunting and a 'Wee Here' sign.

Nightly use of the commode before bed time and the double bed pad strategy thankfully ensured that there were no more early morning, full bed changes.

There was something strangely special and bonding about the joint problem solving of those mini crises.

26

EPA

"Power of Attorney!"

Her Most Wonderfulness very often wakes with sudden declarations.

Disconcertingly, HMW's morning pronouncements very often have consequences for me, as I am quickly roped into addressing an issue that has slipped, unexpectedly into her sleeping brain. But, on this particular Sunday, her early morning sign of life seemed especially unrelated to my reality.

Hooking onto the word 'attorney' I asked, attempting wit, "Do I need a lawyer? Am I in trouble? Are *you* in trouble? Tell me it's you!"

"We should arrange Power of Attorney for Geraldine," HMW explained in a matter of fact manner, which sounded very much as if I should understand her, and she was using the dreaded word 'we'.

I was none the wiser about what it was that Moosh needed, but I was all too familiar with the 'Royal We'. When HMW is intending to take action she uses 'I'. When she uses the Royal We, it means with utter certainty that it will be me who is pressed into action. It is never ever something I had planned and rarely anything that I am intrinsically interested in. (Thinking about it, even when she says, "I", there is often the expectation that I will be involved, as in "I am going to do the garden.")

"What have you got in mind?" I asked, feeling unexpectedly weary - and it wasn't even 9:00am, yet.

"Geraldine is getting too weak to be able to go to the bank with you. If you arrange to have Power of Attorney for her affairs, you will be able to manage her finances for her."

I had precisely no wish at all to be responsible for Moosh's finances. In mine and Ranjit's relationship, it is she who manages incomings and outgoings. I have absolutely no interest, unless she tells me that we need to be scrimping. My earnings come into my account from the city and go to direct debits that I obediently set up, when directed to by HMW She Who Must Be Obeyed. So long as we have money to go on holiday and for the fun stuff, I pay no attention.

I did, however, acknowledge that, although Moosh could make it to the Bearwood branch of Midland Bank with me, her frailty was rendering this difficult and we did find it awkward to manoeuvre her wheelchair within the building.

Now, becoming more fully awake, Her Most Wonderfulness powered up her laptop and requested tea saying, "I'll Google it and show you."

Still miffed that my day was being hijacked, I clumped downstairs to put the kettle on, before checking in on Moosh, whose early morning routine I had already tended to, but who I would soon need to get ready for Mass.

She was happily watching *The Pirates of the Caribbean.* She always got her knickers in a twist watching that film, because her amorous affections swung unfaithfully between Johnny Depp and Orlando Bloom. Today, she was chuntering encouragement to Mr. Depp.

Under the guise of watching the carriage chase, I surreptitiously observed her, mourning the fact that we had reached a point in her life where I was now considering taking over her affairs.

Saddened, I left her to drool over Johnny.

I brought tea and breakfast for HMW and she turned her laptop to me, showing the screen filled with a gov.uk webpage with the title: 'Enduring power of attorney'.

Grudgingly scanning the proffered page, I learnt that what HMW was suggesting was that I be set up to make decisions about not only Moosh's banking, but also her property, pensions, benefits and building society accounts. The site advised that attorneys have a duty to involve the donor, the person for whom the EPA is written (Moosh), and to act in their best interests.

Knowing that family money had caused dispute in more than one set of siblings we knew, I realised that I would need to talk with Aly and Neil, before proceeding to any formal arrangement and possibly before broaching the subject with Moosh.

Heartened that the site was not written in Legalese, I clicked through links to look at a sample EPA form and found that Moosh would need to decide whether, as her attorney, I would have general powers or limited powers. I noted also that there was a time imperative, as EPAs were to be replaced by Legal Power of Attorneys at the end of September, and that I would need to engage a solicitor to act for Moosh.

To her credit, Her Most Wonderfulness knew that finding a solicitor would be far beyond the bounds of my interest, so she volunteered to research in her usual, time proven way: by asking her group of girlfriends.

Rather than procrastinating, I rang Aly and explained what we were considering and that I was not only obligated to inform her but wanted to know that I had her support.

I wasn't overly worried that Aly would object or be concerned, I knew I had her trust, but I was still pleased when she said, "Of course, Al. We know that you'll always act in Moosh's best interests. We should maybe have gone that route while she was with us, but it makes perfect sense that you do so now. Go talk to her."

Grasping the nettle, I returned to Moosh who, by now, was doing her best Captain Jack.

I suggested that we get her dressed for the Doyles and asked her what she would like to wear, joking that a buccaneer outfit might be inappropriate for Mass. With her chuckling mock-piratically, I gathered her camel jacket, cream blouse, black leggings and fresh underwear.

All sorted, I began, "Ma, can I talk to you about something?"

"Of course, Alistair," she answered with the beginning of a quizzical frown. "Is this something serious? You sound serious."

"How would you feel about me looking after your money

for you? And probably your house and accounts and pensions?" I asked, before forging on, "I have been exploring something called an Enduring Power of Attorney, through which you could give me permission to look after your affairs and help you to make decisions and then carry them out."

"That makes a lot of sense," she replied, before asking, "Would I still have a say in things?"

"Most definitely, Ma."

I paused to give what I hoped was a reassuring smile, before continuing, "I don't really want to do it, but I think that it is best to talk about it now, before –"

"Before I can't. Before I lose my marbles?"

Thankfully she chortled. She always covered her worries about what Parkinson's might do to her in the future with humour or direct honesty.

In this instance she covered both bases by adding, "Alistair, I trust you unstintingly. I know that you will do what is best for me. What do we need to do?"

I explained that Ranjit would explore recommended solicitors, who gave good service for women, and that we had time.

"She's good at that, organising," Moosh said, satisfied. "Will we need to go out? A day trip?"

It was my turn to chuckle as I slipped her jacket on and stepped back to check her appearance, "Ma, I don't think we'll be going too far. Not London, or even Birmingham. Maybe just Bearwood. You look good. Let's go wait in the sunshine for the Doyles, before you get ideas about swanning off with Johnny. Or maybe it will be Orlando, today."

HMW worked with characteristic speed, gathering information and opinions from her friends.

Within just three days Moosh and I were heading to West Bromwich, armed with her completed EPA form, in which she had stipulated that she wanted me to have general powers over her affairs, and the identification documentation that we had been told we must provide.

I still had not reconciled myself to this new, unwanted role that we were about to arrange, but Moosh was all atwitter with the excitement of an outing for just the two of us, one that was grander than a wheel around the park or a visit to hospital.

As I helped her out of the car in Astell Park, her eyes lit up at the sight of . . . shops!

At that moment, my stomach growled loudly; I had worked through lunch, so that I would be able to leave school early enough to attend the solicitor's appointment. Staying until absolutely the last possible minute, I was already cutting punctuality ultra-fine.

"We need to get you some food." Moosh observed.

"There's no time, Ma," I countered gently, despite the slight butterflies of tension that were flapping around my rumbling tummy, and focussed away from the collywobbles, concentrating instead on steering Moosh's wheelchair at close to warp speed. "We need to get to the solicitors."

On first meeting, Mrs. Sterling, the solicitor, was an admirable mix of professional, friendly welcome and a cool business-like manner. The entirely mundane, functional office was offset by her presence, a stylishly smart, pinstripe trouser suit, immaculate grey hair and, crucially, a sharp intelligence twinned with a quite startling briskness.

Once we were seated, that briskness was directed entirely

at me, as she opened, "So, Mr. Lanyon, what have you brought your mother here to do, today?"

I had expected the question, but not her tone, so I was a little wrong-footed and hesitant as I explained that my mother would like me to secure an Enduring Power of Attorney, because her Parkinson's was beginning to cause her significant difficulty and we were worried that she may struggle to manage her own affairs.

With practised, impressive speed Mrs. Sterling cast her eyes over the EPA form.

Then her gaze rose to pierce through her chic spectacles, holding me, and her left eyebrow arched enquiringly, "With general powers? No limitations?"

Taken aback at being unexpectedly interviewed, I confirmed that those were my mother's wishes, adding that I had spoken with my sister; that she and her husband were supportive of the proposal and that I understood the requirement to keep records and receipts and that I would be accountable.

"Thank you, Mr. Lanyon. I would like to talk with your mother now, if I may, on her own."

With her eyes, she directed me to the door.

"If you would wait in the reception area."

She stood, lifting her hand for emphasis to shepherd me out, before closing the door behind me.

I was left bristling at being treated somewhat brusquely and I sat, stewing. My stomach burbled to add to my sense of discomfort, as I tried to imagine what Moosh was being asked - I felt faintly criminal.

I was doubly disconcerted when the door was reopened by a now beaming Mrs. Stirling, who invited me in, "Come

Mark, or should I call you Alistair?"

Noting my expression, her smile changed from one of satisfaction to one that was slightly apologetic.

"Forgive me for the pantomime ice queen," she offered. "I have to role play the frostiness to make sure that everything is being done correctly.

"I have spoken with Geraldine, asking whether you are making her take part in this arrangement against her will. Sadly, that happens far too often, but Geraldine is strenuously clear that she trusts you fully.

"More than that, can I say that she is enormously grateful for the support that you have been giving her. And your wife, also. She wanted you to know that. Long may it continue.

"Finally, Geraldine also wanted to clarify that she wants to periodically be able to make gifts, which is perfectly acceptable, but please make careful records of everything. I am certain that you will, but you can never be too careful."

From the moment I re-entered the office, Moosh had been twinkling with amusement at the discomfort I'd been subjected to, but, as soon as we left, she insisted on buying me a consolation Subway, cheekily inquiring, "I do still have some real money don't I? Or am I now like the Queen, and you just pay for everything for me? I think I could get used to being regal!"

Utterly relieved to have navigated the paperwork and the mild, but discomfiting interrogation, I happily suggested that we have a pootle around Marks & Spencer for Moosh's first visit to a retail outlet for almost a year. As I trundled her up and down the aisles, she animatedly looked for gifts for the children, entirely heedless of my vain suggestions that maybe

M&S was not the best place to be buying clothes for teenage boys and a wannabe teenage girl. Determined to buy them something, I managed to channel her to socks (that could be hidden in a drawer) and chocolates (that were expensive, but would make them feel as loved as she intended).

Not even my teasing assertion that I would have to approve her purchases could spoil her shopping delight.

She didn't buy a single thing for herself.

27

The Great Lie In

As we continued to settle into life with Moosh in our house, new routines evolved.

My day started with my and Moosh's pre-school wake up visit and bed check and, if required, bed change. The day drew to a close with organising bedtime, ensuring that the absorbent sheets were positioned correctly, that Moosh was comfortable and a bit of gratuitous, remote control induced giggling, as I raised and lowered, folded and unfolded the bed with Moosh in it.

"You're wicked!" she would howl with hilarity. "Stop or you'll make me wet myself!"

"Better now than in the middle of the night!" I laughed back.

If time allowed, I would watch a bit of telly with Ranjit to numb the brain before sleep and then waking. Over the years of early morning starts for work, my body clock had set itself to fall asleep by 10pm at the very latest: HMW would delight in telling anyone who would listen that I could and would fall asleep anywhere, including in friends' bathrooms or at their dinner tables.

Now, however, getting into bed was the beginning of the last act of the day – the dissecting of the day, Ranjit's sharing of niggles about Moosh, particularly the things that Moosh would not do and most particularly her refusal to accept that, by not asking for help, she was making life difficult for other members of the household.

I have to hold my hands up and admit that, while I hope I presented a well-polished veneer of attentive listening and appropriate support, there was far more than one time when I treated the conversation as HMW's letting off of steam and my brain was already asleep, behind open eyes. On others, wisdom bit my tongue on my observations about the interactions of daughters-in-laws and mothers-in-law.

I was brought up in a family in which, despite only fleeting contact with my paternal grandmother, I was aware from a very young age of the tension that existed every time Granny Lanyon came to visit, or a letter arrived from her, or a phone conversation took place. Granny Lanyon was, by reputation, a harridan, and I have strong memories of my father being sorely vexed by her sniping at his wife. The poorly veiled intimation was always that Moosh's mixed-race blood was an ill tolerated canker on the family tree.

I have, to date, only ever met my own mother-in-law twice, so am extremely unqualified to comment on how I hope I would conduct that particular in-law relationship, but watching HMW and Moosh, and, more especially, hearing about it (on a nightly basis) and to reflect on my position within it, was to marvel at a classic 'rock/hard place' scenario.

Even on her least directive days, HMW would accept that she is genetically wired to be The Boss, to call the shots and have things her way. Scientists have not yet discovered the *Shakti* Gene, the one that underpins female empowerment or *Bossness*, but I can attest with a high degree of certainty that it does exist. As the eldest of five siblings and the first English speaker in an immigrant family, her status of Boss was conferred and strengthened from an early age. So much so that her youngest siblings, both brothers, bestowed upon her the dubious deferential, '*Granjit*' (long before I lovingly gave her that very same pet name, when our granddaughter arrived in our fifties, wittily eliding Granny and Ranjit.)

Inconveniently, Moosh was at a point in her life when, by virtue of mine and Ranjit's marriage, she believed that she, too, had a rightful claim to the queenly throne of Bossness in the Lanyon household. She knew with the brightest diamondlike clarity, from her own decade of having a dragon mother-in-law, that a degree of power lay in her hands; the capacity to assert status, to expect to be listened to, to have influence. In even more crystalline form (from the long-lost Indian dimension of her young adult, pre-marriage life in Malaya) came the knowledge that, as an (Anglo) Indian mother-in-law, the mother of a son, in her relationship with Ranjit, she was The Boss. At some deeply hidden level, I think she quite liked this, although, as far as I could intuit, she never really pushed it – but maybe I speak as a loving, and therefore blind, son.

That left me in a household with two Bosses and me.

As an Indian daughter-in-law to an Anglo-Indian mother-in-law, Ranjit's social rearing dictated that she must be dutiful and deferential, and, to be fair, she did try to be. She was attentive and thoughtful and continually ensured that Moosh's needs and wants were met, buying the items that she required, generously supplemented with treats that she knew Moosh would relish. At the same time, in her own house, where she had previously been the undisputed Boss, she expected an increasingly frail and dependent Moosh to respond to her well-intentioned guidance, particularly as it was given for Moosh's own good, to keep her safe from harm.

Moosh, on the other hand, was vested in a steely, determined resistance, wrought through hardship. Having lived, from a very early age, away from her birth family in the care of nuns, she was never inculcated in the ways of family life. This situation was not improved by having had a husband who was, by his own admission, mystified by womankind. Despite clearly being besotted with her throughout their marriage and being her staunchest ally in the in-law friction with his own mother, he frequently treated her harshly. As a result, she was an armadillo of self-protectiveness and a lone she-wolf who would have been perfectly content to live outside the boundaries of family, had grandchildren not arrived and her health allowed. She expected to do exactly what she wanted, how ever well-meant Ranjit's lead was.

It is most fortunate that Ranjit and I had long since had our last child, as HMW's nightly venting about Moosh's quiet refusal to be told** (** 'guided by a concerned and dutiful daughter-in-law, who is only trying to do the best for her') rendered it certain that no more children would be added to our family.

The thing that gave Ranjit by far the greatest contraceptive bedtime headache of all was that she plaintively ended each recounting of Moosh's single minded refusal to comply with her attempted steering by saying, "But she does what you ask her to do: I am only the daughter-in-law."

If I had not valued my life so highly, or indeed my dangly bits, I might have countered by cautiously suggesting, "Maybe it's the way that I say it."

Having a strong self-protective streak of my own and still harbouring some lustful hopes for the future, I never did give voice to this thought. More importantly, I knew that Ranjit was right: Moosh, for whatever reason, did not listen to her in the same way. The irrefutable truth was that the only person under our roof that she was inclined to pay any heed to was me.

The ramifications of Moosh's non-heeding were sharply illustrated on the evening that I was stopped early in a Senior Leadership Meeting by a call from Ranjit on my mobile phone.

I am not great at being interrupted by home, when I am in full-on professional mode. Neither am I keen on the constant interruptability that mobile phones have brought to our modern lives, so I was mortified that it was my phone that was ringing.

Seeing the caller ID and being tuned to fear the worst, I was a mixture of worried terseness at the intrusion and embarrassment that it was my phone that was ringing, melded with naked fear, so my, "Yes?" in answering was, at best, gruff, but I don't think Ranjit heard it.

"It's Geraldine!" she declared, alarm erupting from the phone in my hand. "She's on the floor and we can't move her!"

The faces of my team immediately mirrored my concern. Elaine, mouthed, "We'll go. You go."

As they tidied and stood to leave, Ranjit continued, "She's in her room, between her bed and the chair. I don't know where she was going. I've told her, haven't I? 'Just call me or ring the bell.'

"But no! And now she's on the floor and we can't move her. Arun is strong enough, but he's not home from school yet. I can't. And Alex can't. And we can't even manage it together. She just won't listen to me!"

I waited for a gap in the anguished torrent to interject, "Do you need to call an ambulance? Did something happen? You know, inside her? Her head? Her heart?"

The exasperated cascade of frustration began again,"No! She wanted to come to the kitchen, because I was making food!She said that she stood up, turned, lost balance and did her 'drifting to the floor thing!' I have put a cushion under her head and Alex and I are next to her, but we can't move her. I need you to come home."

And so, I hastily left the school where I was nominally in charge and arrived home, where The Boss Of Our House was feeling desperately unheard, unlistened to and disregarded.

Entering Moosh's room, the offender was exactly where Ranjit had said, prone on the carpet. Ranjit sat on the floor next to her on one side with Alex on the other trying to make himself helpful, but clearly frustrated that he had not been able to lift his Grandma.

Moosh looked mightily chuffed by all the attention and I swear she visibly preened when I asked her, gently, "What have you been up to this time, you monster?"

"One minute I was going to the kitchen, the next I was drifting to the floor," she voiced from the carpet.

"They couldn't manage to pick me up, but you're here now," she added, entirely unaware of or unconcerned by the worry on Alex's face or the frustration radiating in palpable waves from Ranjit.

"Your world famous 'drifting to the floor' trick? Checking on the carpet again?" I chided, but keeping my tone soft. "Let's see if we can get you up. I'll need you to help me a bit."

To further pulses of now furious frustration from Ranjit, Moosh complied with my guidance, allowing me to raise her shoulders and carefully push her into a seating position. Between the two of us, she and I raised her knees, so that her feet were flat on the floor. Ranjit stared in disbelief, as Moosh pushed down on her feet to help me to raise her enough to slide a foot stool underneath her posterior, and she almost exploded when Moosh pushed for all she was worth, as I lifted her from the stool to a standing position. Moving quickly to her front, as she stood wobbling, but independent, allowed me to hold her hands and walk her backwards until she could sit back down in her chair. I could no longer see the look on Ranjit's face, but I could sense her glaring eyes lancing into my back.

I managed not to crow or to visibly polish my Golden Son halo, or even to look at Ranjit.

Instead I opted for, "I know that you like going on your adventures, Ma, but we really wish that you would call for help. It is much easier to help you to walk than to get you up off the floor. My old man's back isn't up to lifting you and Ranjit had to call me out of a meeting to come to help. Next time, if you are not hurt, I think Ranjit should just make you comfortable on the floor and wait until I come home."

With that, Ranjit stalked into the kitchen. Alex hung around, visibly distressed by his inability to help Moosh up.

I made space for him and he edged in, putting his hand on her shoulder.

"Please let us help you, Grandma. You had me really scared. And I thought I could lift you, but you are heavy for someone so tiny."

"Charmer!" she chuckled, looking up at him, before patting his hand and saying, "I'm sorry for worrying you."

"I think it is Mom who was most worried," suggested Alex.

"I'm sorry, Ranjit," Moosh called, genuinely apologetic.

There was the resounding clunk of a saucepan on the hob, but no answer, so I walked gingerly down the corridor, unsurprised that Ranjit was staring back at me from the middle of the kitchen.

As I approached, she pointed in the general direction of Moosh and stage hissed, "She helped you!"

Her eyes shone with impotent tears.

"I tried! We both tried to help her up! She'll do whatever you ask, but she just won't listen to me. The Golden One walks in and it's, 'Oh yes, I'll help you! You just tell me what you need me to do.'"

I pulled her to me, clumsily trying to wipe her cheeks and hug her at the same time, "I'll talk to her again, later. I'll try to get her to cooperate with you more."

It is possible that I should have paid greater heed to the warning signs.

28

Moosh's House

Moosh never lived in her house again.

From her second major incident, she went first to Aly's, then to Brotton Hospital, back to Aly's and then to ours. Despite all the efforts by Sandwell care services, once she had lain in the bathroom for over two days, I could never bring myself to countenance her going back. The risk was too great.

There had been a brief moment, when I visited her in the ward in Brotton, in which she had mooted the idea of going home, even suggesting that she would be happy for carers to support her, but it was only a brief flicker of a moment: romantic rather than realistic. She loved that house. It was Dad's gift to her: the house that he had bought for her, calculating that it was close enough for Aly and I to look after her, when he knew that he would not be alive to do so himself.

For the first ten months after she left the house, I would visit Shakespeare Road weekly to collect post, discarding the junk and sifting through for any correspondence that required a response and anything from Moosh's circle of friends that would brighten her day.

On my post visits, I also attempted to keep her plants alive. I moved the more fragile ones to our house and promised myself that I could give enough care once a week to keep cacti, succulents and orchids thriving – thank goodness she had such a liking for plants which require less water. Her triffid-like spider plants and her Mother-In-Law's Tongue and her Money Tree were impossible to kill, and I became very fond of them for helping me to look as if I was doing a decent job of tending them.

Very early on, I worked through her larder, fridge, freezer and food cupboards. It was fortunate that Moosh's digestive system had always been of a cast-iron constitution, as I found food stuffs that were over twenty years past their use by date: they would already have been well out of date when she transported them from Shrewsbury - in the late 80s.

Far from being mortified, when I reported this to her, Moosh was insulted that I was in any way concerned, asserting (quite correctly), "Well, I'm here aren't I, so no harm was done!"

She was appalled that I had thrown almost everything away without giving her the right to veto my intent.

There were occasional forays to the house to collect furniture and keepsakes to create a Moosh space, first the grand one at Aly's and then the more modest one at ours. As a result, her home was increasingly denuded and over time became more of a storage space.

Despite its diminishing contents, there were other forays at Moosh's behest, when I would be dispatched by her to collect something that she needed, and that she knew was still there. On those occasions, her memory was laser sharp, allowing her to direct me to the precise section of the correct drawer to locate the particular item she wanted, recalled from her internal inventory. I marvelled that, in her brain, where memory was more and more often a challenge, she retained this ability.

Once the decision was made that Moosh would move from Aly's to ours, what to do with her house became a refrain in our conversations and in discussions between Ranjit and me.

I wanted to sell the house. It had no emotional significance to me. It had never been my home. I never once slept there, nor did I ever once have a meal at the dinner table there. To be honest, I never much liked it, covered as it was in Artex on every single surface that could hold the 70s' favourite decorative surface. To me, it represented a burden, as keeping an eye on it was just one more plate for me to spin, at a time when I was deep into a build project at school and anticipating another inspection - I always seemed to be expecting an inspection. Lastly, an entirely irrational part of me blamed the house for the fact that Moosh had had her two major collapses there.

Ranjit was on the fence, trying to fact find and calculate what impact selling the house would have on accessing future financial support with care.

Moosh was clear: the house was not for sale. It was her home; the only one that she had ever been truly able to settle in; the one that she had lived longest in; the last gesture of love from the husband she had moved from pillar to post, across the globe and all around the UK, to follow.

After fourteen house moves in twenty-four itinerant years of marriage, it was Dad's final gift to her.

I respected Moosh's wishes and would not sell without her permission. What I did suggest to her was that this was an ideal opportunity for me to enter the property development field. In doing so, I could remove the datedness of the décor, and make the house more liveable, so that when Aly and Team Loftus came to visit her, they could stay there. I was scrupulously honest with her that this would put us on the front foot, should she decide to sell in the years ahead.

Wonderfully, she was rather excited about this approach.

I set to with gusto.

Firstly, I cleared the house in a most unforgiving declutter. In so doing, much clutter was sent to further clutter Aly's cluttered house. Precious items were checked with Moosh, with her either asking for them to be stored at Aly's or mine or for them to be accepted as early bequests.

In this way, my grandmother's dining table and chairs and Moosh's camphor wood chest came to our house. I had loved each of them from boyhood, as it had been my job to polish them for almost as long as I could remember. Moosh knew that I associated the chest with her and the table with my Dad and that I intended to treasure them. I also took out the living room door, with its stunning stained glasswork, hoping to find a doorway at our home that would properly showcase it.

At Moosh's insistence, Aly had already taken our grandfather's magnificent longcase clock and other beautiful pieces of personal significance, when Moosh had moved to Woodlands.

Beyond the sentimental, useful items were scavenged by both households: beds, chests of drawers, sets of shelves, crockery, cutlery, storage boxes, tools. To this day, when I do woodwork, I use tools that it was my responsibility to oil and keep rust free, while my father was abroad in the 80s: sometimes, when I use those tools, I feel as if I am working with him, in spirit form, at my shoulder, checking on the care and skill of my endeavour. Our kitchen cupboards and our mobile home in the Languedoc boast indestructible and highly serviceable Tupperware that is as old as me, which has previously been to Yorkshire, Germany, Cyprus, Germany a second time, Dorset, Lincolnshire, Essex and Shropshire.

Boot loads of pictures, furniture, books, miscellaneous items and some very questionable music CDs were donated to churches and to charity shops. Despite my initial energy, the declutter took weeks.

Once the house was cleared of belongings, I had a moment of horrified self-flagellation. I was standing in Moosh's empty house taking in the condition of the decoration and the fixtures. Almost nothing had been touched in the nineteen years that she had lived there: the same living room carpet with its huge swirling pattern of browns, oranges and white; the same aluminium framed patio door to the garden, which I was appalled to discover was entirely unlockable; the same electric fire in the hearth that had never worked; the electrical wiring that was out of date; the bathroom where we had found Moosh, that was so cramped as to be barely useable; the Artex.

A lava flow of shame burned through me. I berated myself for never trying to improve the condition of Moosh's house while she lived in it, yet here I was, developing it, knowing that she would, now, *never* live in it. I consoled myself that I had offered and urged many times, but Moosh's independence was fiercest when keeping her home as her very own and she would change things only as they suited her.

Following the clearance, one could truly appreciate the full range of that Artex. Some people maintain that, at the height of its popularity, Artexing was an art form. I do know that a friend's brother became prodigiously wealthy from setting himself up as an Artexer at the height of its demand in the mid-80s. I have long had a hankering to learn the skill of plastering, to be able to work through the steps from prepping the wall, applying PVA and then a first coat of plaster, before skimming, smoothing and second coating and finally the bit I truly admire: the polishing to a glass smooth surface. I am certain that applying Artex requires similar skills, but I can never see it in the same positive light, because of Moosh's house. If one were ever to perversely create a Museum of Artex, akin to the admittedly wonderful Musée de la Porte (Museum of the Door) in Pézenas, Moosh's house could have provided examples of dozens of ways of using the medium. Walls and ceilings were coated in it, so too were the chimney breast, the side panels on the bath and many of the doors, indeed the bedroom doors had framed panels of Artex swirls on both sides. It took weeks to remove just the miniscule amount that I managed, before I admitted defeat. I carted the doors and bath panels to the tip, together with anything that I could remove from the house that was decorated in it, but eventually I needed help and arranged for it to be cleared. I can say, hand on heart, that I never want to see Artex again.

Our friend, Glen, took care of almost all the physical work, removing the accursed Artex; moving a wall to slightly increase the size of that bathroom; moving a doorway; liaising with electricians and plasterers and preparing for all of the finishing.

Through the whole process Glen and I deferred to Moosh as the client, so I brought her catalogues of kitchen units and bathroom suites; samples of carpets, underlays, vinyl and kitchen and bathroom tiles; paint colour cards and match pots.

Moosh was delightedly energised by the project and she and I had hours of fun in her room at our house, discussing options with the voice of numerous TV property developers in our heads, reminding us to keep things neutral and not to put our own preferences into the house, but provide a blank canvas for a future owner.

Once the discussions were complete, I always abided by Moosh's final choice: well almost always - on a whim at B&Q, Glen and I ditched Moosh's preferred bathroom stipulation in favour of an absolute bargain set that was sleek but ridiculously cheap. We never admitted this to her.

Mindful of cost and wanting to have a hand (or at least a finger) in the development, I did everything that I could find time for and that I felt confident in, which was mainly destruction (ripping out the carpets and unwanted fitted cupboards) and final touches (painting each room, reinstalling doors and basic furniture, putting up curtain rails etc).

Once the carpets were in (a neutral beige) the focus shifted to the garden.

Moosh loved her garden and, for a tiny woman in her

spritely sixties and then her slowing down seventies, she had singlehandedly developed a stunning shrubbery with an impressive array of beautiful planting. In its pomp it was a thing of splendour, having something to catch and please the eye on every day of each season.

With Moosh having been absent for almost a year, the garden was a tangled snarl of climbers and creepers and rampant, verdant foliage. I hacked and pruned and strimmed, imagining that I was David Bellamy hunting through the undergrowth. I unearthed the derelict pond that Moosh had never managed to have restored and with regret decided that it could not be rescued, so filled it in. I could then trim and snip and mow to reclaim the former shape that Moosh had created in the layout of the borders.

I went up to Moosh's bedroom which overlooked the back garden to survey the progress and was forced to admit that, again, the task was beyond me. There was a whole extra patch, beyond Moosh's ornamental garden, which she had rarely ventured into. It was where the previous owner had housed his dogs and looked to me to be the size of a small paddock, filled to almost chest height with nettles and brambles and other invaders.

I arranged for the O'Reilly brothers to come to do the necessary and they arrived, just two of them with a wagon and enough tools of garden destruction to arm a small country. Either their worn features were indicative of the twosome having endured hard lives or the boys were a good ten years older than me, but they were rock solid, built like brick outhouses and there was nothing that they could not shift. After just one afternoon of vehement *feck*ing, there was not a nettle or unwanted privet standing, no slabs or concrete chunks or shards of glass or tile, just a surface ready for turf to be laid on to become a 'family lawn' in future house vending particulars.

The project was most challenging for Ranjit.

While I had the benefit of feeling useful and could see the fruits of my labours and argue that my efforts were saving us bits of money here and there, Ranjit was left to be the primary carer for Moosh. Every second that I spent at Shakespeare Road came out of non-carer time, when I was supposed to be part of the team around Moosh. I was at Moosh's more than at home for chunks of the Easter holiday, weekends and evenings after school.

Despite my entreaties to Moosh, each time I left to go to work on her house, she only really paid lip service to them. On several occasions I would find myself up a ladder or deep in undergrowth trying to free my hands to be able to answer my phone, already anticipating that I was about to be called home, Ranjit having reached the end of her tether and needing me back at the ranch to do my turn of Moosh wrangling.

Ranjit tried to be patient but I swear that there was sometimes devilment in Moosh's shenanigans, while I was away trying to spruce up her house. When I would return home, there was often an amused twinkle in her eye.

Taking Moosh to see her house was a bittersweet experience.

Ranjit came with us (possibly to see what her sacrifices equated to). I was proud of the way the house looked and knew that every one of the team who had worked on it had delivered. I knew, too, that it was marketable, should the need or opportunity arise. I remained, however, riddled with guilt that Moosh had never lived in the modernised comfort that it now offered.

I need not have worried.

From the moment we arrived on the small drive with the now neatly trimmed fuchsia shrub, she was effulgent. I guided her up the step that had caused us so much worry a year before, me walking backwards, her following my feet. She admired the carpet and marvelled at the Artexless walls and positively swooned at the effect of the patchwork of tiles in the kitchen, coupled with the new units. She insisted that we went upstairs to see the bathroom that Glen had built and so I sat her on the second step and lifted her and backed her onto the step above and then again and again until we safely reached the landing.

"Oh my, that is a big improvement! It feels so much bigger!" she gushed. "But is the bedroom tiny?"

We checked the smaller bedrooms before ending in her old room. She was both shocked and impressed that it still felt a good size.

Her bedroom gave her the grandstand view that was one of my primary angsts, that of her beloved garden, but, again, I need not have worried.

As she peered out over what had been her pride and joy, she beamed, "Oh yes, this is fabulous! And thank you for keeping my favourite plants. They look magnificent! And the lawn looks super. It's taking well, already."

She turned her face up to mine, resplendent with pleasure and gratitude in equal measure, so that she could fix her gaze on me as she said, "Thank you. It really is wonderful. You've done a great job."

And then she added, "But I could never live here: it's too modern for me. We'll just keep it for a little while, so that Alyson can stay here."

As I bumped her back down the stairs on her bottom, I felt like a schoolboy who had just shown his Mum his school report and been patted on the head for good effort. It was a wonderful feeling.

Ranjit, who had been our quiet companion on the exploration of the house, ceding the cloak of Bossness to Moosh in her home, caught my eye as I checked that Moosh was safely strapped in and mouthed, "It's fabulous."

Double Gold Star!

We kept the house.

29

The Emergence Of Alco-Moosh

One of the unexpected changes in Moosh, when she came back from her stay with Aly, was that she had developed a liking for a drink before bedtime - not an Ovaltine or a hot chocolate, but an alcoholic bevvy!

Moosh had never been much of a drinker.

I always thought that this was a conscious decision rooted in her convent-instilled sense of propriety and reinforced by the fact that Dad was a habitual and not always pleasant drinker. During her married life, a glass of Asti Spumante on a special occasion was enough for her to feel that she was pushing the boat out and buying a bottle Mateus Rose was the height of sophistication, possibly because it was exotically Portuguese or because she was taken by the flattened, flask shaped bottle.

In my childhood, towards the end Dad's army days, our Sunday afternoon routine was to visit the Sergeant's Mess *en famille* for a pre-roast dinner relax. Moosh would always ask for a peppermint cordial that I have never seen since.

Before taking a sip, she would already be a little heady and feeling naughty, even though, with all of the lemonade, the diluted alcohol content must have been negligible.

Possibly my first ever tastes of alcohol were her offering me illicit sips from those Sunday lunchtime peppermints, allowing me to join in with her own daring forays into alcohol intake, stage whispering with an impish wink, "There's just a tiny bit of something in there."

As I grew into my teens, drink became her enemy, with Dad's drinking becoming heavier. If she joined Dad in the pub, she would, as often as not, choose a soft drink or limit herself to just one glass of something only mildly alcoholic.

She had good cause to be afraid of Dad's drinking, as he could range from maudlin to unpleasant to aggressive to violent when drunk. My two earliest memories from our time in Cyprus, when I was between three and five years of age, are one joyous one of searching for snakes in the *bondoo* (scrub land) with Aly and a pack of Mowgli-like three to seven year olds; and a traumatic one of Moosh and I leaving a tiny Aly asleep, alone, in our army quarters to go to search for Dad, who had not come home from a stag night with his army mates. We found him in a ditch, physically unable to move, when roused from his drunken inertia, but still capable of a torrent of cruel, misogynistic invective.

Moosh carried both visible physical scars and emotional wounds from Dad's moments of uncontrolled, drunken lashing out.

Years later, I came to understand the desperate pain and self-loathing that drove his drinking, which he shared with me in one startlingly enlightening afternoon of searing honesty, recounting horrific acts committed in combat

213

including a dreadful final act of friendship, which broke his heart and continued to haunt and traumatise him years later. On that afternoon, the same day as he begged me to be a better father than him, he sought absolution from his teenage son, absolution that I was unqualified to give.

To his dying day, he continued to attempt to wash that pain away, on every anniversary of his friend's death and on almost every other day. He never succeeded, but I never saw him sober after 2:00pm from the day I started to take notice, at the age of thirteen. Moosh frequently implored me to intercede with Dad to ease off on his drinking, but, knowing the source of his pain, I believed that to be an impossible conversation to have.

So, he drank.

Once Dad died, Moosh became a little more relaxed around drink. She could let go in family celebrations where we had drinks on the table and appreciated that Ranjit always thought of her taste preferences when choosing a fizzy wine for a special occasion. She would even allow herself more than one glass. However, I never once saw her worse for wear due to drink in all the years of my childhood or young adulthood, or in the years that she lived, independently, in the house that Dad bought for her, when he knew that, through his hard living and hard drinking, he was seriously ill and did not have long left.

Against that backdrop of her abstemious life, I nearly keeled over with shock the night Moosh asked, "Do you have any whisky in the big blue cupboard?"

It was a Sunday evening and she was engrossed in *Lewis* and I had just enquired whether there was anything that I could get her, thinking maybe she'd like a cuppa or a biscuit.

"Ma, when on Earth did you start drinking whisky?" I mocked.

She was an amusing mixture of feigned nonchalance and perky naughtiness as she quipped back, "I've decided that I like the taste, and life is too short to not have little treats." Then she capped it with, "Besides, it never hurt your father."

"Well, actually, it's what killed him, wasn't it?" I shot back, a tad stunned at her light-hearted reference to Dad, which I took to be borderline insensitive.

"Oh, I didn't mean anything nasty. It's just that I never thought of drinking it while he was alive, because I was so cross with him, but I often had a whisky and coke at night time, in Loftus with Alyson, and I realised that I'd been missing out, because I didn't want to encourage Daddy," she explained.

Slightly mollified by her conciliatory tone, I responded, "I'm certain that I can find some whisky left over from New Year's Eve, but I think we are all out of coke. I'll pop down to Global and get a bottle, if you like."

"Oooh, would you? You are my knight in shining armour! Thank you!"

She was genuinely delighted.

Back from the off licence, I rooted out a moderate assortment of unfinished bottles from soirees dating back years and from visits of whisky loving friends.

I went through to her, quite proudly, to report the menu on offer, but she said, "Oh, you choose. I have no idea what Alyson gave me. It just warmed me up and got me ready for bed."

So back I went and poured a modest measure into her lidded drinking cup, thinking how comical it was to have Moosh drink alcohol through the spout of what looked like a baby's beaker. I topped up the beaker with coke, sniffing it before heading back. I have never come to terms with whisky, but it smelled just about palatable to me.

I was filled with a sense of filial pride in my waiter service, which was immediately punctured, when Moosh sipped and grimaced, "Did you put any whisky in? Alyson makes them much stronger than this!"

"Blimey, Ma! You'll fall asleep before Inspector Lewis has his first clue!" I warned in mock-offence, but went on, "Slurp a bit and I will add a bit more whisky."

She chortled as I headed back to the kitchen and then called all the way down the corridor, "Don't be mingy!"

And, so, a pattern was set for the months ahead. Sunday nights, before bedtime, I would settle Moosh down with her treat of a whisky and coke.

I sometimes pondered whether the whisky should be drunk, while she was on her truck load of medication, but, in her words, "Life is too short."

For her, in her 80th year, there was a sense of liberation, shaking of shackles of the proprieties and stays of her younger self, coming out of the shadow cast by the drinking of our Dad and just a little bit of sticking two fingers up at her illness, (although she would never, ever have raised two fingers in real life).

It is only in recent months that I have learned that Moosh had a few other allies, who she would inveigle into supplying her with an illicit whisky. On our Sunday evenings, it was her treat. On other occasions she just wanted to have some, because part of her always saw it as being just a little daring and naughty.

Fair play to her, I say!

30

Alex's 18th Birthday Party

Alex's eighteenth birthday fell nearly three months after Moosh took up residence at our house. Our first landmark event for several years, coming a fortnight before our twentieth wedding anniversary. There was always going to be a party. It was always going to be big and it was always going to be loud.

In our household, big parties were always held at the Bear Tavern. The function room upstairs holds around 150. In those days, we could squeeze in a few more at a quiet push.

Parties are the preserve of Her Most Wonderfulness; she whirls herself into a frenzy of excitement and planning, for which there is a coefficient in the amount of stress generated and nagging emitted. Of course, to her it is not nagging; the communication of requirements is simply her thinking through her to do lists out loud. Despite years of me asserting, with varying degrees of forthrightness, that her out loud to do lists soon become my actual to do lists, nothing has changed.

We will be walking to the pub or sitting on the bus and I will be thinking about any one of the myriad things that buzz through my head, when, out of the far distant left field, with absolutely no preamble, will come, "Photoboards! We should go through all of our photos and make big boards of photos of Alex."

That's how it was, one Sunday morning, when I had gone back to bed after completing Moosh's breakfast and bedding routine, probably hoping for a few minutes to day dream about a holiday away for just the two of us or, much more likely, something Sunday-morning-lustful, when HMW said, "She won't be able to come. Will she?"

Shifting my brain back from wherever it was, maybe a walk in Beddgelert in early summer sunshine or some sultry, wanton behaviour, I started to file through anything that might equate with *she*. The majority of our friends are women. There's my sister, four sister's-in-law, our daughter, several neighbours and over fifty percent of our friends.

The randomness of *she* and the tumult of possibilities now swirling around my brain led me to ask with some annoyance, "Which *she*?"

"Geraldine. How are you going to tell her that she can't come to Alex's party?" she illuminated me in a way that was a perfect example of why I love her so much: a) no preamble; b) stressing on a Sunday morning; c) creating a problem; d) passing the problem to me.

"Why am I telling her? Why aren't *you* telling her?" I demanded, before taking the necessary thought step backwards and asking, "Why can't she come?"

"It will be too noisy for her, won't it? And it won't be safe to take her up and down the stairs, will it?" (Assertions that clearly expected my agreement.)

"And she won't want to stay all night. And you won't be able to drink, if we take her." (Trying to clinch the non-argument with threats of curtailed enjoyment.)

I felt myself rising to unintended bait, "Have you decided this already, or is it up for discussion?"

"Well, I'm right aren't I? It will be very noisy. She won't be able to get up or down the stairs. We won't be home until well after midnight. And she's not good with crowds." HMW fired.

Without warning, this was now an argument, from unpre-saged spark to conflagration in milliseconds.

"Mum will love to see Alex play and she would hate to miss his party. I'm not telling her that she's not coming. If you want to tell her that you don't want her there, then feel free." I challenged.

"I didn't say that I don't want her there," was HMW's feeble, albeit accurate, defence. "You tell me how we can do it. How do we get her there? You tell me how to get her there safely!"

There it was: HMW's mulling was now my problem to solve. I like to think that, with all hopes of rumpy-pumpy obliterated, I huffed off out of bed with some level of decorum.

In our house, the lead in time for planning any event is relatively brief. We are not exactly lastminute.com, but we do plan and organise things quickly. Suffice it to say that, despite agreeing for three years that we would one day marry, HMW and I planned, organised and celebrated our wedding in a seventeen-week time frame – before spreadsheets were a thing AND for less than £1000 including honeymoon, to boot.

Whatever other whinges I may have (and there are many) we do get things done.

HMW's challenge left me with three weeks: three weeks to co-ordinate a solution to a problem that I had not seen. I would need to confirm that Moosh did indeed want to be at the party with a live band and close to 200 lairy revellers. I would then need to practice stairs with Moosh. There was also the issue of Moosh's bedtime.

Most days of the year, I am very grumpy if I am not in bed by 10:00pm and, ideally, I'll be snoring by 10:05pm. At weekends I can, with sufficient warning, stretch this to midnight, but I'd actually prefer not to. So, the option that immediately appealed to me was to take Moosh to the party, navigate the stairs, stay until 10:00pm and then slope off with the entirely valid reason of Moosh needing her bed, with multiple Brownie Points for being the Perfect Son.

The not insignificant drawback to this solution was that HMW would almost certainly remove my dangly bits with a very blunt knife, should I dare to suggest that I not be around to fulfil my tidying away chores and help to carry the PA equipment back down to the car park and supervise her own ziggy-zaggy walk home.

Another solution was clearly needed.

Moosh did indeed want to come to the party!

She looked shocked that anyone could have thought she might not. Not wanting to put any pressure on their daughter-in-law/mother-in-law relationship, I claimed that

221

the query was mine (Brownie Point). Moosh and I started to practice assisted-stair-climbing on the stairs at home. It is a surprise that both of us lived.

We tried and failed the strategy of Moosh walking up in front of me, clinging to the banister, with me behind her to ensure that the only way that she would tumble was forwards (although, of course, she could have fallen backwards onto me).

This morphed into a very brief attempt at assisted-stair-crawling, but Moosh could not achieve sufficient leverage to raise herself up the stairs. Instead, she slid backwards, with me trying to block her, eventually kneeling behind her and crouching over her, holding the stair rail with my left hand and pushing my right against the wall and her forehead against the carpet. Despite the precariousness of this position, we were both in hysterics.

Our best success was achieved by replicating our me-backwards-you-forwards Loo Run walk, with me walking backwards up the stairs and Moosh lifting her feet to follow me. Interestingly, her movement was more fluid than on the flat, but we were both worried by the fact that I was holding her weight by gripping her forearms and agreed that neither of us wanted me to be questioned for bruising her. We decided that this was a three-man/three-person job: we needed a catcher or a back-stop.

Getting down was easy. We did the Bum-Shuffle, one step at a time with me in front of Moosh, facing her to arrest any slide: it worked each time, but we were both a little concerned about what party-goers and members of the public would make of a nearly-eighty-year-old coming down a flight of pub stairs on her rear end, although we both expected that more than one other person would do the Bum-Shuffle on the night - it was an 18th birthday party after all.

So Moosh was going to the party and we knew how to get her upstairs and down again, albeit ungracefully.

Unexpectedly, Moosh suggested what would be the eventual solution to the bedtime problem, "Why don't we ask Florence whether she would be willing to do some extra hours? She could collect me from The Bear and bring me home and you can get on with the party. I'll be fine with that."

You could have knocked me out of a very tall tree with a tiny feather from a juvenile robin's bottom, but it would have taken an even tinier feather to knock down Her Most Wonderfulness. The stunned disbelief on her face was a picture, but she was relieved that satisfactory solutions had been found without her having to get involved and quietly delighted that Moosh could come after all.

Guardian Angel Florence readily agreed to the extra hours, but asked that we make it a private arrangement. She was delighted when, without her even asking, I doubled the agency's hourly rate. This led to a short-lived dream of me appointing her, privately, as a full-time carer, but I could not afford it and she needed greater job security than the hours that I could offer.

On party night, I drove us all down with final bits and pieces in my trusty Zafira, plus Moosh and her wheelchair. I wheeled Moosh through the downstairs bar in her party finery with her waving regally to everyone we past, unaware that they were not coming up to the party in the function room.

We had a minor wobble as we climbed the stairs. Moosh managed the long first flight, before having a momentary loss of strength on the landing by the loos, so I bodily lifted her up the last short flight and gingerly lowered her into her wheelchair, realising that I had foolishly tweaked my back.

The party itself was fabulous, other than Aly having to turn round at Sheffield with Liam and Jess and heading back to Loftus. They were all heading off to Gran Canaria in the morning and she was too exhausted to drive down, show her face, turn round and head home before being up early to go to the airport: six hours of driving for one hour of party made no sense. Alex's eighteen-year-old friends were great fun and a huge credit to themselves. The forty-somethings could not be quite so proud of themselves, as the expected lairy behaviour abounded raucously in their age group. Alex's band, Knock Door Run, played an excellent set, in what turned out to be their last ever gig. Very importantly, Moosh had a riot of a night, being surrounded at every moment by a steady stream of well-wishers, several of whom offered her a drink and were only slightly taken aback when she requested a large whisky and coke.

Just before her wheelchair turned into a pumpkin at 10:00pm, a slightly squiffy Moosh bade her farewells and we made for the stairs. I had asked for any willing helping hands in guiding her down, worried about further tweaking my back. My involvement was unnecessary as one of Alex's muscly mates lifted Moosh into his arms (as if she weighed the same as that robin's feather) and carried her all the way to the bottom. I almost had to physically unlock her arms from round his torso, as she was swooningly smitten.

I wheeled Moosh up the road, followed by the strains of Knock Door Run booming through the windows, and handed her over to Florence at the corner. They set off up the road with Moosh recounting the evening through whisky-infused euphoria and doing her very best to sing the chorus to one of Alex's songs.

As it was, despite my confident predictions, no one did the Bum-Shuffle, but my deputy head, Shirl, had to be tended to in the Ladies by a swarm of eighteen-year-olds.

She had arrived for the night, a vision of loveliness twinned with her young daughter in eye-catching black and white polkadots, only to catch the eye again later, having succumbed to a spectacular bout of alcohol induced illness just short of the toilet stalls.

Shirl was also involved in the best recorded memory of the night, thereby catching the collective eye for a third time. Ever the one to know how to do things better (she would call it being helpful), and always in the thick of everything, Shirl took over videoing duties, certain that she knew which shots would be best and where to get them from. Shirl is a climber, whether it is onto a stage or up onto tables to dance in restaurants.

And so it was that Shirl had, now very much worse for wear, found herself perched on the three inch deep back rest of a wall-fixed sofa to gain the best vantage point from which to video the band. I can only imagine that she believed that she, too, was bonded to the wall, possibly with static electricity. In a moment that is now part of our family folklore, Shirl drunkenly lost her mural attachment and gently peeled away from the wall.

Alex's friend, Mountain Man, from whom Shirl had only recently wrested the video camera, saw what was happening and, left with the choice of 'catch the falling, drunk lady' or 'catch the expensive camera', heroically chose the latter. The video is a wonderful record of the band being filmed in landscape, giving it their all, and then an almost perfect arc, described by Shirl's fall, followed by an imperceptible jostle and blur and then back to landscape, as Mountain Man took over filming duties, all within the span of a couple of beats of the song.

Shirl didn't feel a thing and her pride was only temporarily bruised.

Guardian Angel Florence laughed to me later that, in between mildly inebriated, attempted renditions of Alex's choruses, Moosh told her about being carried down the stairs by her young hunk *many, many times*, before finally falling very contentedly asleep.

It was one of her great nights.

31

The God Box

Moosh had always been an avid reader.

Novels, magazines, newspapers and catalogues were always a feature of each of our homes. *The Pears' Cyclopaedia* was her go to source of information, updated annually for most of the years of my childhood. Every month the *Readers Digest* would arrive and sit on the occasional table next to her chair until it was fully thumbed. Whenever we were living in the UK, *The Express* (Daily or Sunday) was delivered each day. She favoured historical fiction, when reading for leisure, but was always armed with books about gardening and nature.

As her children, Alyson and I were owners of our own books from as early as I could remember, when, despite scrupulously scrimping and saving to budget the house keeping from our father's army salary, she regularly allowed us to buy books as treats. Each birthday and Christmas would bring annuals and encyclopaediae and *The Guinness Book of Records*.

Now ensconced in her room in our house, the very same occasional table stood, well-polished, next to her wingback chair with a small mountain of the same type of tomes.

With her enforced sedentary lifestyle, reading and television were her most accessible pastimes. *Readers Digest* was now delivered to our door, but I refused to have *The Express* delivered, arguing, possibly unfairly, that her years of faithful, unquestioning reading of it, fuelled most of the differences in our opinions and asserting, only slightly in jest, that if she ordered it, I would make sure that it went straight to the recycling box. Added to her old favourites were prayer books, her missal and, incongruously, stacks of glossy, gossip magazines. She had always had her prayer books in our homes, but now they were kept close at hand. When I quizzed her about the glossy magazines, she simply cackled.

On top of her reverently stacked pyramid of prayer books was a small, red charity collection box and with it a tiny pair of scissors. Next to the books was a plethora of pens. I think that I inherited my love of pens and all things stationery from Moosh.

Although the collection box was clearly emblazoned with the word 'missio' surmounted with a cross, Alyson, Ranjit and I always called it *The God Box*.

To my knowledge, Moosh is the only person, either Christian, or of any other faith, to keep a God Box, but she did so for years, long before she moved to us. Although I do not recall it being in Shrewsbury, while my father was still alive, when Moosh moved to Shakespeare Road, it had lived on the Malaysian walnut coffee table, the same table that I once drilled through in an attempt to refit a batten - I had silently dreaded my father finding the evidence of my botch job up to the day he died. The God Box had not been on that table in Shrewsbury, but it was a fixture in Oldbury and it travelled with her to Alyson's in Loftus and then to our house.

Despite her love of a naughty joke (not lewd, but risqué) and her capacity to unexpectedly erupt into ribald mirth at something that you knew was just wrong, Moosh was, at heart and certainly in the depths of her soul, a profoundly pious person. The God Box was testament to her devotion.

Moosh was Roman Catholic to her core. Her faith gave her great comfort and strength but her interpretation of it had perplexed me from a young age, despite my own attraction to the Church.

In my pre-teens, I had been confounded when, on our two-mile Sunday yomp to Saints Peter and Paul Church, we would always walk on the north side of Skellingthorpe Road only until we reached St. Helen's Avenue. Every week, without fail, we would cross to the south side until we were opposite our Church, where we again crossed the road to go inside to dip our fingers in holy water, make the sign of the cross, genuflect at our pew and take our seats. After we had done this for many weeks and were again on our way to Mass and approaching St. Helen's Avenue, I queried the crossing of the road, to which Moosh turned eyes filled with contempt towards Holy Cross Church and kept walking.

Holy Cross was an Anglican Church, very much the wrong church, apparently.

My youthful sense of tolerance must have been affronted, because on the return journey, I challenged Moosh more directly and suggested that maybe she was a religious bigot (I was twelve and seemingly brave). What followed was a forced march home and a stony silence, Moosh's ultimate sanction, which lasted for 48 hours - a world record for me being in the doghouse. The thing that I found most unfathomable was that the forced march had taken us back to the house where Moosh's Anglican husband was waiting for us and photo's of Moosh's much loved Anglican father-in-law hung in pride of place.

From that early age, I had known that Moosh's piety could easily take on, what seemed to me, a puritanical edge. One example of this was the way she was scornful of many of my father's favourite female singers. Admittedly, they were frequently very revealingly clad, as was becoming more and more in vogue in the 70s & 80s of my youth. I distinctly remember Moosh loudly huffing out of the room when Tina Turner appeared on TV in a short dress, rocking out as only Tina can (silver and tasselled, if I'm not mistaken, the dress). I knew that scanty = improper = bad = Godless, particularly if Dad was nearby: Suzi Quatro, not scantily clad but leather-sheathed and low-zipped, had a similar effect in fuelling Moosh's ire and bringing forth menacing mutterings about Godlessness . . . and the less said about Cher the better!

Somehow, I escaped censure, despite my testosterone-fuel led, teenage fondness of the lingerie sections of Moosh's ever present stack of catalogues. The closest I came to chastisement for Godlessness was when Moosh returned my copy of Wilbur Smith's *The Sunbird*. Not a word was said and it was only some years later when I was reorganising my books (alphabetically by author and then by date of publication, obviously) that I realised that the previously nubile, naked woman adorning the spine was still nubile, but now sported a carefully drawn bikini, courtesy of Moosh, the self-designated censor of Godlessness. Thinking back, I had noticed other tastefully modest examples of Moosh's artwork over the years, usually in her own *National Geographic* magazines.

The God Box was Moosh's very personal embodiment of her quiet campaign to ensure that respect was paid to God. At some point after her move to Shakespeare Road, she took to methodically snipping out every typing of the name of God that she came across in every newspaper or magazine that she handled. She never articulated why she did this, but I can see a logic to her not wanting God's name to be put in the recycling bin to be discarded. Every fastidiously cut out *God* was placed in The God Box. She never told us what she did with them when the box was full, but she must have filled it many times over from the day she first started, because she somehow managed to continue to manipulate her tiny pair of scissors long after arthritis put a stop to most other activities.

Adding further to the time consuming demands of her campaign was the capitalising of *god* to *God*, before the word was carefully snipped and stored. Her pens were always ready to ensure that proper respect was afforded to God. Her glossy magazines were her prime target for editing, as, much as she enjoyed reading about the royals and celebrities, she was indignant at the editors' omission of capital Gs. In this regard, even library books were not beyond her pen: she would never snip a *God* from a library book, but she would determinedly capitalise those Gs before the book was returned.

I am certain that I must sound as if I am mocking. I am not.

While I never understood Moosh's take on her faith, nor the particular devotion that caused her to keep on filling The God Box, I was in awe of that faith and enormously grateful for the strength it gave her, particularly in the most difficult years of her life.

32

The Search

Despite our desire to be her last home, it was very quickly clear that Moosh residing with us was not a forever solution.

Each of us had, however, derived different thresholds.

Ranjit's was very much duty bound: 'This is what we are supposed to do and we must flex our lives to make it happen, unless that is no longer doable'.

Moosh's was, if Ranjit and I reached a point where our skill level meant that we could not manage to care for her. She was also very clear that she did not want our looking after her to disrupt our care for her grandchildren, which, in her mind, included us continuing in our current jobs, so that we could maintain the same level of comparatively comfortable lifestyle for our children.

My own threshold remained as it had been when I spoke to Aly in the lead up to Moosh's move to Woodlands: I wanted to continue until Moosh could no longer recognise me. I knew, beyond doubt, that I would struggle emotionally with caring for Moosh if she did not know who I was and we were unable to interact as son and mother.

When she was still living at Shakespeare Road and we were having conversations about where and how might be safest for her to live, Moosh's opening gambit was that she never wanted to be involved with social workers or carers and, most adamantly, would not entertain any form of home for the elderly. She wanted to live independently or to die trying.

In all of the conversations that led up to Moosh coming to live with us, between Ranjit and me, myself and Moosh and the three of us together, the actual threshold, or rather the tipping point, was left entirely undecided. None of us had anticipated that Moosh coming to live with us would put enormous pressure on mine and Ranjit's marriage. How naïve!

Ranjit uncomplainingly embraced all of the tasks required to make Moosh comfortable. She laundered, she cooked, she made countless drinks, she monitored medication, she helped Moosh on Loo Runs, she popped in, she chatted, she researched, she shopped, she bought treats. She did all of these things added to her daytime teaching job and alongside all of the other tasks that were already in her remit as mother and wife. She took all of that in her stride, willingly and with full acceptance. It was how she had expected her life to be from an early age.

I helped as much as my job allowed. Prior to Moosh's arrival, I would have been working a 60-70 hour week, spiking to 100 hours in mad weeks like School Reports Checking Week. Even with hospital visits after each of her falls and trips to Loftus after she left hospital, I managed to keep on top of work. Mine and Ranjit's relationship had always been based on us sharing chores, so I generally cooked at weekends and did my chores from shopping to tidying to hoovering, whatever got us through life. At weekends I went with Arun to his football matches, which was a highlight not a chore, but it was still time that had to be found. Just as for Ranjit, once Moosh joined us, I just factored her in, adding what she needed from me to my list for the day or the week.

We knew that our new arrangements would not last forever, but, while we were setting up Moosh's room in late January and early February, full of our shared sense of purpose, we had talked about giving Moosh stability for 'at least five years'. Again, naïve.

The tipping point was not the added 'lifeload' of what Moosh needed from us. It was that daily niggle of Ranjit's that Moosh would not do things at her bidding in the way that she would for me. Just as on the day that I raced back from my meeting at school to lift Moosh from the carpet, our life was becoming characterised by instances of, 'She'll do whatever you ask, but she just won't listen to me'.

Ranjit would never have made it an 'It's me or the dog' situation; I was never forced to choose. However, her almost daily distress at being unheeded and her involuntary anger at me that Moosh would listen to me always put me in Moosh's camp. To Ranjit, I did not have to side with Moosh, I was simply part of the pair of people who inflicted unintended wounds by virtue of Moosh responding to me alone. Ranjit never directed ire at Moosh; she just vented her pain at me.

We found ourselves in a pressure cooker of Ranjit's carefully compartmentalised hurt and anger and my impotent 'What would you have me do? She's my mother!'. Without ever expecting to, we acknowledged that our marriage was in danger.

There was no last straw, no explosion, more a widening chasm of unhappiness. I realised, one Saturday in mid-June, that I was losing Ranjit; she was silently seething and unreachably distant.

We had nothing thought through, no alternative agreed and certainly nothing in place.

That is not to say that we had not looked at homes or spoken with Moosh. Helpful conversations had happened and Moosh and I had searched, in preparation for an accepted future need. However, I was struggling to satisfy her criteria. There were only two, but I had been unable to meet them: a) close to us & b) a Catholic care home.

Soon after Moosh joined us, she and I had visited St. Joseph's in Harborne. It was less than two miles from our home and Catholic from the foundations to the roof tiles, being run by The Little Sisters Of The Poor. I knew that it was home to at least one of the teachers from my junior seminarian boarding school and to many nuns. It also had enviably wonderful ratings. We had been told that the waiting list was long, but, undeterred, Moosh wanted to go for a visit and so I made an appointment.

Upon arrival, whilst I was disappointed that we were not walking through billowing wafts of incense, the Catholic ethos was all-pervasive, and convent-raised Moosh felt instantly at home. She adopted her most beatific expression as we were escorted around the building. I was quietly certain that she regretted not bringing her rosary beads and missal and maybe a nun's wimple to fully convey how seamlessly she would fit in. The drawback was that, even through her rose window glasses, it was very clear to Moosh that she was a good two decades younger than most of the residents that we saw. When I spoke privately with our escort, she was very sympathetic to Moosh's wishes, but expressed apologetically that Moosh was simply not sufficiently infirm to secure a place. I considered trying to play my old school tie through the network of Birmingham clergy, but that was never my style.

I drove Moosh home full of regret.

Ever since, a residual Catholic part of me has believed that, had I been able to secure Moosh a place at St. Joseph's, she would have piously and contentedly lived out her remaining days and quite quickly made her way to her God.

Over Easter, Ranjit and I had headed away for a previously planned few days.

There was no way that I was going to ask Aly to come to cover for us – it was just too soon, after all of the pain, for that to be a possibility. We needed to access a respite placement. From her list of care facilities, Moosh's social worker suggested a home that she had high regard for, which offered much of what we needed. It was fairly local, in a part of Birmingham that I was very familiar with. It was never going to measure up to St. Joseph's, but Moosh was committed to Ranjit and me going away and was adamant that she was willing to spend our long weekend away at the recommended home, but I wanted to be sure, so I took her to visit.

Whereas the atmosphere at St. Joseph's was instantly homely and devout, the respite home was clinical and almost hospital-like. It boasted an impressive array of activities for its residents, but, unfortunately, one of these, a music session, was in progress in the residents' lounge immediately on the left as we entered. Moosh discernibly shrivelled, a snail doused in salt, her spirit retreating within her invisible shell, her face a mask of resignation.

I leant close to her ear and whispered, "Let's leave, Ma. This is not for you."

To my amazement, she replied with unexpected strength in her voice, "No. You are going for your trip away, and I am going to be alright here."

We completed the formalities and left quickly with the manageress calling behind us, "We'll see you in a few days, Mrs. Lanyon."

As I was buckling her into the Zafira, Moosh took my face in her hands, which were icily cold, and said, "Just this once for your respite, but promise me that I will never come here again."

I promised.

33

In The Parish

After Easter, working from the list provided by her social worker, Moosh and I had continued to visit homes, feeling no immediate pressure, despite an extended period of frailty. At that point there had been no insurmountable alarms, we were just jointly planning for the longer-term, while Moosh felt vital enough to provide input.

We arranged to visit a care facility, in a neighbouring part of the borough, that had been home to a friend's father. I wheeled Moosh into the home and we were shown around by Karen, a kindly member of staff. Her welcome exuded unaffected warmth and she was a rich mine of information. Despite not being at her strongest, Moosh was giving positive nods and asking interested questions.

Having completed the tour, we returned to the office where a large aquarium instantly captured Moosh's fascination as she started to name mollies, guppies, swordtails and gouramis. Capitalising on the diversion, Karen asked Moosh if she could have a few minutes with me to go through some further administrative details. Moosh readily agreed, her eyes following a small but vivid shoal of neon tetras, and Karen suggested that we step outside.

"I'm very pleased that we were recommended to you, Mark, and Geraldine is a gem," she started, "but I am afraid that there may have been a misunderstanding."

At my confused look, Karen continued with impressive sensitivity, "I think that Geraldine's needs are beyond the parameters that we are able to meet. I know that today is not one of her stronger days, but, from your description of her current requirements, I am as certain as I can be without her medical records, that she will need to be placed in a *nursing* home. Mark, we are only a care home."

We spoke a little more, with Karen urging that I contact Moosh's social worker for clarification. She went through my list of prospective homes, identifying other care facilities on the list that she believed would be unable to meet the needs that she believed Moosh now presented.

Speaking with Karen was simultaneously dispiriting in opening my eyes to the deterioration in Moosh, and enormously supportive in giving me immediate steps to take.

To her credit, Moosh's social worker was very proactive, apologising immediately that the rapid deterioration in Moosh, since her last review, may mean that the documentation did not reflect her current needs. We agreed that I would arrange a further meeting with Moosh's G.P. and consultant.

A fortnight later, armed with an updated report of her needs and a new list of prospective nursing homes, Moosh and I visited two homes out towards Dudley. Moosh was still engaging in the search with an encouraging positivity. In our minds we were still thinking long-term, medium-term at worst, still with no immediate pressure and no sense of the looming clouds.

Both had good reviews. Both presented as well organised. The staff at each in turn were welcoming, friendly, knowledgeable and were reported to be skilled in supporting residents presenting with Moosh's set of needs. The first had links with a church, not Catholic, but a church. The other was surrounded by gardens full of shrubs and borders full of vibrant, nodding blooms. Moosh balked at both. She was not hostile in any way, but her body language in each was defensive, more so in the second.

Resigned to another unsuccessful visit, I wheeled Moosh to the car and helped her up and in. She was initially resistant to my enquiries as to what was troubling her and remained unreachable as we drove down the long dual carriageway back towards Birmingham.

It was only as we turned off the Wolverhampton Road, up towards the water tower that stands guardian-like on the hill above Warley Woods, that Moosh reached out for my gearstick arm and said, "I'm sorry Alistair. They are just too far away. I can't expect you to drive that far every time you come to visit. It's not fair."

"But, Ma, if you like one of them, if you trust them to look after you, we will drive for however long it takes to get to you," I reassured her, gratified by her thoughtfulness.

As we headed down the hill to home, we agreed to give it time and to ponder. I promised to search closer to home, and she promised to try to weigh up the benefits of either one of the homes against her expressed desire not to impose on us.

That had been early May.

By mid-June the dynamic had changed drastically, and Ranjit was struggling. She knew, intellectually, that I was not taking Moosh's side against her, but, emotionally, she felt isolated in her own home.

I needed to act, before our marriage imploded.

I am not sure what I believe about fate, but I do believe in people. It was a person who was the key to me deciding that I had found a home that might work for Moosh.

I was not looking for a home on the Thursday night that I was driving home from a school governing body meeting. I was exhausted and not actively thinking about anything, just listening to the radio and allowing my subconscious to get me home. Possibly as a result, I did not take my intended late route home, but found myself driving up Bearwood Road from Smethwick and spotted Bearwood Nursing Home on my right. I am certain that I had never really noticed it before. Almost without thinking and despite the hour, I turned into the car park and, on spec, rang the bell.

Through the glazing, I saw a young woman in a blue uniform approach, smiling.

She let me in and said, "I was just passing and saw you. I don't recognise you. Who are you visiting?"

Slightly blearily, after 13½ hours at work, I explained, "I was just passing and I thought I'd ask . . ."

She smiled, expectantly, as I searched for the next part of my sentence.

"You see, my Mum has Parkinson's and is very poorly," I stumbled on my words, suddenly overcome.

She guided me to a pair of comfy chairs, saying, "My name is Sabina. I am one of the carers. Are you looking for a place for your mother?"

At my nod, she continued, "Several of our residents do have Parkinson's. We also cater for people who are suffering from dementia. You will need to talk to Mrs. Sandhu, but I am sure that you could do that quite quickly. I can take you down to the nurse's station so that you can arrange an appointment."

It was only a few short sentences, but the friendliness of her welcome, her intelligent receptiveness and the warmth and kindness that Sabina showed me all convinced me. At our school, I was always proud when visitors commended the welcome that they received from our front of house staff. For me, it spoke volumes about us. Here was a young woman, who I had momentarily called away from heading off to her next task, and yet she found the time to allow me to fumble over my words, quickly ascertain what I needed, give me appropriate advice and reassure me.

I was sold.

When Moosh and I visited on the Saturday morning, after I had made phone calls on the Friday and checked through the reviews of the home with Ranjit, I was nervous, but Moosh was positive.

I was worried that the home had no links to a church, was directly on the main road, did not look out onto greenery and seemed very large in comparison to most of the others that we had visited. I had a very positive feeling about the place, but without wanting to do it any disservice, we had been to grander ones. I was, also, a tiny bit anxious as to what Moosh would make of a home with a predominantly Asian staff – I could never tell which way her mixed-raceness would swing her thinking. She had said nothing that gave me any insight into her quite jaunty demeanour.

As we pootled around the home, Moosh was far more interactive with the staff than I had witnessed in any of the other homes, so my worries on that score were unfounded. She quietly dismissed the residents' room, but showed real interest in the room that would be hers, if she chose Bearwood Nursing Home. She asked about what she could have in her room and whether it would be permissible for us to bring her favourite chair from home, even joking that it was her lucky Scrabble chair.

Even with everything going so positively, I almost fell over when Moosh declared, "Yes. I'll take that room. Thank you."

She did not even confer with me, just came out with it.

With assurances made that the home would contact the social worker to move the process forward and with me still in shock, Moosh said that we could go home now, her decision made.

It was only in the car, as we drove home, that I was able to ask, my questions becoming a rapid jumble, "What just happened? What made you decide on this one? How did you decide so quickly?"

She chuckled, "It is simple. This is on your way home from school, so it is easy for you to visit me. It is close to home, your home, the home that you have all made me welcome in, so Ranjit and the children can visit me, too. We have not been able to find a Catholic home, but this is in the Oratory parish, so the priests will be able to visit me here, if I can not get to church. Plus, it is not far from Shakespeare Road, so you can take me there, if you don't mind, so that is an unexpected bonus. Even if you can't take me, I will feel close to your father, which is important to me."

And there it was.

This incredibly poorly woman, who was deteriorating rapidly and who I thought of as withering away, who was, on an alarmingly frequent basis, unable to speak coherently, had puzzled it all out for herself and decided what was best for her. On the inside, obscured by all the befuddlement that we saw from the outside, she was as sharp as ever.

I marvelled.

I still do.

34

The End Of Life Plan

As Moosh had settled with us, we had moved to the centre of a new network of support around her, replicating the one that had been established at Aly's: a team in which we and Moosh were the only non-experts, the non-professionals.

There were carers visiting every day; occupational therapists providing advice and resources as required; a social worker gathering information and signposting us to avenues of support; consultants and G.P.s monitoring Moosh's Parkinson's, arthritis and other ailments. And there was us: not really having a clue. That might be doing us a disservice, but just as when you choose a builder or a roofer to carry out works on your house and they are the experts who can speak in jargon that can leave you bamboozled, we were very much at the centre of a network in which every other person knew more about what could be done than we did.

All we knew was Moosh . . .

but now I had to advocate for Moosh in meeting after meeting.

This often made me reflect on how I was in a position that was a complete reversal of my role at school, where I was the lead professional: it gave me a sharper insight into how our parents must often feel. Clearly, each professional who was supporting Moosh, came from their service with a set of guidelines and policies that they were to apply and operate within. I have operated with parallel guidelines in education. At school, it was the parents who were unfamiliar with the jargon, the policies, the criteria. It was they who often felt on the outside of the decision-making process. It was they whose lives were inextricably bound with the needs of their children. And it was they who carried on living with the challenges of their lives, after we had done our work and gone home.

As a head teacher in meetings at school, particularly those about our children who needed the greatest support, I was often impassioned, emotional and even tearful, as we tried to improve the circumstances of children's lives in order to give them greater chances of safety, stability, happiness and success. Nevertheless, the truth was that, however much I felt invested in the cause of any of our children, however much we angsted about them during the weekends or holidays, they were not actually directly connected to me or us at school; even at our well intentioned best, in their lives, we were fleeting passers through.

Sitting with Moosh, at the centre of the team that had been built around her, on one level it was fascinating to observe how professionals in other walks of life operate, to learn about the frameworks within which they worked. However, at all times, I was on the receiving end, gauging their effectiveness to ascertain how much help they would be to Moosh. In this network, it was they who were the transient ones, and we who were left when they had given their input.

I went into Moosh's first round of meetings bolstered by advice from John, but I also took my experience of being part of similar meetings in a school setting. My headteacher experience gave me a degree of confidence. I knew that I was adept at marshalling arguments to make a case and at ensuring that others were persuaded by my argument. Despite being the non-expert in the room, I was confident that I would be able to make a robust case for Moosh regarding funding or care arrangements.

That is not to say that the meetings were easy or straightforward, far from it. As the non-expert in the team, I was always talking to people who knew the systems they were operating in far better than I did. This necessitated research and phone calls to ensure that I understood the criteria and parameters, so that we were asking for the right things at the correct times.

A little later in Moosh's time with us, another meeting was being held to decide what level of funding Moosh was entitled to. I felt that Moosh was in danger of her habit of careful saving being used to offset the amount of funding that she would be allowed. I had been asked to pull together all of the information about Moosh's finances: her different income streams from Dad's army pension and her own state pension, set alongside the savings that she had frugally accrued. I knew what Moosh's bank account looked like. I knew what she stood to earn from the sale of her house, if we ever got that far. I argued strenuously that Moosh's frugality and my scrupulous care of her bank account should not be counted against her in reducing the allocation of funding.

I felt a keen affinity with those parents of children with special educational needs who I had supported to try to ensure that their children received the support that they needed, which always came with a financial cost.

The fact that the outcome of that meeting was that Moosh was indeed granted the maximum funding for the next period of time, has not diminished my sense of non-expert embattlement and powerlessness, despite the passage of years.

Sometimes it was Moosh who made those meetings challenging, just as Aly had complained in January.

In the days leading up to the very last meeting held at our home, Moosh had been in alarmingly steep decline and the prognosis from her doctor's was bleak: he used the warning phrases 'palliative care' and 'weeks not months'. The move to Bearwood Nursing Home was in process, but we were once again fearing the very worst and expecting that we would lose her in the next few days, without her ever needing her place. So grave was my concern that I had considered asking for the meeting to be deferred, thinking that it would serve no purpose if, as seemed likely, she passed away. Deciding, on balance, to go ahead, I had phoned the chair of the meeting to warn her that Moosh was very weak. She was full of understanding and promised to keep the meeting as brief as possible and assured me that, although she would like to see Moosh, Moosh would not be expected to take any active part in the meeting.

Suffice it to say that I was very nearly struck dumb when Moosh put in her best ever impersonation of Lazarus to greet the chair warmly, somehow hoisting herself out of her wheelchair to offer a hug and answering the few questions asked of her with a display of spryness that had me internally shrieking, "Ma! You were dead less than twenty minutes ago!"

Although I did manage to keep the scream inside my head, the chair quietly registered my dumbfoundedness, resting a placating hand on my arm, letting me know that, just as Aly had been told before, she had witnessed this behaviour before.

At the end of that last meeting at our house, after I had wheeled Moosh back to her room and just before the other professionals departed, the chair said the twenty words that possibly shook me the most in all of the time that I spent with Moosh as her protector, "*Mark, I think that it might be time for you to think about an End of Life Plan with your Mum.*"

Her words were full of care and concern, but they tore through me, eviscerating.

I knew that Moosh was gravely ill. Intellectually I knew that she was, once again, close to death. However, having another person, someone who I had deep respect for and who I knew had Moosh's best interests at heart, talk about end of life, shifted my world into stark focus.

Seeing their impact, she quickly went on, "I am not saying that Geraldine is going to die imminently, but you know that we are in a phase of palliative care. While she is able to talk with you and express her feelings, it might be good for you and for her to capture her thoughts about what she would like to happen as things move forward."

I must have continued to look puzzled or pained or both, because she added, "You do not have to think of everything yourself. There are some very helpful documents or frameworks that you can use as starting points. You can then adapt one to work for you and Geraldine. Once you and Geraldine have made a start and you have a good idea of what your Mum's wishes are, you can share it with the nursing home and add to it or change it as appropriate. I know that you and Geraldine talk a great deal, so I am certain that you already have a lot of this information."

Throughout the entire cycle of meetings that I was involved in for Moosh, I always felt that we were being well supported and that the professionals in her team were genuinely striving to make things as good as possible for her. Frequently, I was absolutely certain that the arrangements put in place for Moosh were the most generous interpretations of the rule book possible, sometimes flexing the limits to Moosh's advantage in a way that I would be proud of, had I been doing the same for a child at school.

Moosh and I could not bring ourselves to physically write down her End of Life Plan. She mithered that doing so made 'it all' seem too much like preparing for the blade of a guillotine to fall, and I was all too willing to duck out of the finality that formalisation in written words implied. However, over the course of just two days, we did talk through every element of several model plans, so that I was fully briefed on all manner of things that were important: how she wanted to be treated in the nursing home; who she wanted us to inform when she passed away; that she would like me to keep taking her to Mass for as long as possible from the nursing home; who had been provided with copies of her updated will; how often she would like her hair done; that she wanted Father Guy to officiate at her funeral; that she wanted to be buried with Dad; that Aly knew where the cemetery documents were kept.

As you would expect, some of the talk was sombre and heavy, but, despite her frailty, Moosh rallied to share her thoughts and sometimes we howled.

Despite agreeing that a nursing home was now the most workable option, Moosh was still prone to bouts of ambivalence and worry, so she stunned me when she said, "While we're talking about how I'd like to be looked after, there is one thing that I'd like you to do for me at the home . . ." (taking a pensive inhalation of breath) "my toenails."

I must have looked horrified, because Moosh started to snort with laughter, "No, not you! It's bad enough that you've learned to glue my teeth in and cream my bottom, but I could never ask you to go near my feet. They need special tools to deal with my toenails - like sheep shears."

"But they never seem to grow?" I queried, which only made her hoot.

"The girls do it for me, when you are all at school. There are some things that I couldn't subject you to! I asked the carers to do them for me and they are lovely about it."

I'm sure that I had never once expressed distaste at Moosh's feet, but they were as arthritically knobbly as her hands and surmounted with toenails that made the horn of a quinquagenarian rhino look like the most delicate Delft china. Seeing my naked relief sent Moosh into a paroxysm

252

of glee. It wasn't exactly life and death or even end of life, but it certainly relieved the pressure.

Through those conversations, one thing remained un-equivocally constant and one thing surprised me when it changed. She reminded me of what I had known for years: the most important thing to Moosh was that, if she looked likely to die, I must ensure that she received the Last Rites – again. Her feelings about resuscitation, however, had completely changed: she no longer wanted resuscitation, should that discussion ever come up again.

At least I would not get that particular decision wrong next time.

I would never have been brave enough to start that series of conversations with Moosh. In truth we had covered many elements of it in our chats in the garden outside Sheldon Block at City Hospital, but, thanks to that gentle steer from the chair towards an End of Life Plan, I knew much more clearly what Moosh wanted.

It would not make what happened any less painful, but knowing Moosh's wishes allowed me to navigate with greater confidence.

35

Compassionate Leave

Moosh continued to be visibly weakening, almost before our eyes. We were being told that she had, with a fair wind and God's help, perhaps three weeks to live.

I still did not have the heart or emotional strength to formalise the End of Life Plan in writing, but we agreed to go ahead with the move to the nursing home to secure round the clock professional care, and set the date for the Saturday after my birthday, so that Moosh could celebrate one last birthday with me.

I requested compassionate leave from the chair of the governing body at school. I was entitled to three days, but, ever supportive, he suggested that I take the week to spend time with Moosh. I leapt at the chance.

I had no qualms about leaving school. The build was approaching completion. I had proudly taken the staff across to visit the new building, which was very clearly taking shape as a school, although some wag, possibly Carole, suggested that it could equally pass for a new hospital, or more worryingly, a very plush prison. We agreed that, while it was not perfect, it was an enormous improvement on what we would be leaving behind, where rats scuttled from beneath our terrapin huts, that had been temporary for decades, and brambles grew up through the floor of the Year 1 classrooms. There were excited conversations about how we could capitalise on the potential offered by different spaces.

We would be moving in after the summer holiday and, with guidance from the local authority, had agreed a closedown packing period at the end of term, followed by an unpacking and set up period in September. I had applied the suggested formula for calculating the number of packing cases and come up with a total of 750, which would be delivered in the last full week of term.

There was an outside chance that we would be inspected before the end of term, as our last inspection had been just over five years ago. Very few teachers or head teachers will ever say that they enjoy inspections or look forward to them. There are better times to be inspected (when results have been good, and data is strong, and the school is settled) and there are worse times (at the end of the school year, when everyone is trying valiantly to hold the wheels on). Our data showed that our children were making progress, but we were on our knees, focussed on the move and crossing everything that we would be given the time to wow the inspectors in our shiny, new school. As a token gesture to inspection readiness I asked staff to jolly up displays in the corridors, and accepted their quiet grumbles that these would be taken down in a fortnight. They would not; they would still be fresh on the boards when the old school was demolished.

To salve my conscience at leaving school, I took home all 400+ children's reports and the school's self-evaluation form, planning to spend the very early mornings working and the remainder of the day doing whatever Moosh chose for us to do. I was determined to minimise the creation of additional work for other staff that me prioritising Moosh might cause. Looking back, I can not pretend that this was wise, but hindsight is powerful and rarely generous.

Moosh was delighted that I had asked for compassionate leave and when I told her that I had been granted a full school week, giving me nine days to devote to her, including my birthday, she was effusive in her gratitude, repeatedly checking that I had expressed my thanks, and hers, strongly enough to the chair of governors and staff at school. Despite her frailty of body, she was predominantly sharp of mind and quickly realised that for much of those nine days she would have me all to herself, everyone else would be at school or college. I was mildly astonished that she was sensitive enough not to articulate the joy of this in front of Ranjit. My astonishment was magnified when she refused my suggestion that I cancel the carer visits a week earlier than her move. She countered that if the carers continued to support her until we settled her into the home, I could work uninterrupted, allowing us more time to do enjoyable things: she had a list.

To most people the list was mundane in the extreme; to Moosh it was all she wanted.

We mounted an expedition to Safeway, the supermarket on the high street, allowing Moosh the unimaginable excitement of simply being out in the world, surrounded by people, with the super-bonus of being in a wheelchair, which doubled magnificently as a ramming tool in crowded aisles. She caused havoc, Boudicca in her dotage imperiously commanding her charioteer between the trolleys of other shoppers in search of green bananas, biscuits, chocolates and toiletries. Feeble at home, she found the strength to reach for items on shelves, her head close enough to crotch height to cause significant alarm for unwary customers. When I hurriedly steered her away, simultaneously mouthing my apology to a particularly discomforted woman and hissing a warning to Moosh, she hooted her delight.

Her seated position caused me all manner of challenge. Most distressingly, it put her at the same level as children in their pushchairs. She adored little ones and would greet them, coo at them and generally shower them with affection. At the till, I had Moosh's chair in front of me, while I placed her shopping on the conveyor belt. A mother had her little one in a pushchair, while she was packing her items away. Moosh found herself facing the little girl and went into her befriending routine. Seeing an attentive, friendly face, the little one happily entered into the game, but squeaked when Moosh reached out to pat her cheek, just as her mother was paying for her purchases. With my head teacher head on, I was horrified that Moosh's actions might be seen as in any way predatory. With furiously burning cheeks, I shamed myself by becoming one of those people who apologises for the innocent behaviour of their elderly relatives. I quietly hated myself.

Not yet finished with her shenanigans, outside the supermarket Moosh realised that her position put her almost face to face with a magnificent Great Dane, who, unbeknownst to its owner, she was communing with. Ever since I was a child, outings with Moosh were prone to elongation due to her habit of entering into long and meaningful conversations with almost every animal she passed: dogs, cats, horses, canaries, budgies, koi in a pond; only Yorkshire Terriers, Chihuahuas and Jack Russells were immune, being dismissed as yappy annoyances. I caught her trying to slip the Great Dane half a bar of Bournville, which she had managed to surreptitiously unwrap. I was bemused that her body seemed to pick and choose when to give her full access to her fine motor skills and rued the fact that this no longer happened at helpful times.

Together, we packed up her room.

Or, at least, she directed, and I wrapped and boxed. From her significantly shrunken array of belongings and treasures, we decided what would remain at our house and what she could fit into her new room. Her shells and corals and her eggs would stay with us, together with the treasured family tree, the collection of pottery pieces that she had made and the occasional tables inherited from Granny Lanyon's house. Some of her coats and hats and scarves would stay in her little wardrobe and the alarming fox fur scarves (again from Granny Lanyon). On the "nursing home" list, alongside the small pile of boxes were her footstool, one of her beloved wingback chairs (there was no space for both), her Zimmer and her wheelchair.

She looked bereft that her life, represented in the things she had space for, was constantly being whittled down. I too was saddened that, yet again, the horizons of her world were shrinking.

In a moment of dark reflection, she commented, "I may not even need these for very long."

Seeking to lift her spirits, I suggested that we look through some of the mountain of photographs in albums, and loose ones and slides that we would keep safely for her. I asked her to tell me about the family holidays that were captured in purpling pictures: Girvan, where, climbing a hill above the town, we bumped into two ladies who had known Granny Lanyon; Penzance where Dad had surprised us by walking us to Lanyon Manor in the tiny village of Gwinear; Tresco in the Scilly Islands when I remember Moosh and Dad being at their closest.

Moosh came back to herself when she chortled through the memory of Dad sending me off to participate in the "manly pursuit" of lobster potting on a stormy sea on that holiday in the Scillies, tears pouring down her cheeks as she recounted my green tinge when I returned, having lost my stomach to the sea, only to find Dad gleefully tucking into a truly mighty *Homarus gammarus* in the hotel restaurant.

Prompted by more photographs, we reminisced about the school holidays from our boarding schools, when Aly and I had flown to Iran to join our parents in the only post-army home that we ever truly shared and where we had visited Roman and biblical sites and wild camped next to remote waterfalls and seemingly swanned from one expat party to another. There were albums depicting trips to Turkey and Canada and the Holy Land with dear friends, which took her off into smiling, misty eyed reveries, and others of mine and Aly's childhoods, which she stroked silently.

I scorched my way through the children's reports by rising

at 4:00am and working through three sets, proof reading the first few in detail to gauge the level and type of errors, then skim reading the rest, making notes for the teachers of any changes to be made or rewrites required. I always thoroughly enjoyed writing a short, personalised comment to the child, before signing off on their report. Every July, Ranjit took me to task for the hours that these comments added to what was already a time-consuming hill in the end of year, work mountains, but I always told myself that it was what the children deserved after all of their efforts during the year. The early start meant that by 10:00am the rest of the day was Moosh's to direct and by Wednesday I was able to drop the reports off at school to be finished off, copied and enveloped ready to be sent out to parents; one more task completed.

On Wednesday afternoon, Moosh asked if we could go to visit her house to have a last look around and to pick some flowers from her garden. Fortunately, I had popped in since our last visit to run the mower over the lawn and have a quick prune of the shrubs, so I knew that the garden was ready for inspection and the house was still sparklingly welcoming in its pristine, post-refurb newness.

As we drove, I made Moosh promise that we would not re-enact our bottom shuffling up the stairs and to my relief she agreed. I picked up fish and chips and little plastic forks from the corner and then wheeled Moosh through the house before helping her to step down to the garden from the kitchen. I sat on the kitchen step, while she cradled her packet on her lap, and we basked in the warmth of the sun and the flowery abundance that she had spent her happy years creating.

After eating, I pushed Moosh a few metres further to the edge of the patio, from where she could instruct me to snip roses, geraniums and aquilegia to gather into a handsome bunch. She had already emotionally separated herself from the house. In its freshly decorated state, still infused with the odour of its recently applied paint, it was no longer her home. Leaving her garden, however, was a test that I was fearing.

But Moosh surprised me by smiling, "It will be good for someone else to enjoy it and tend it. Please keep it looking beautiful, until it is time to pass it on to them."

I spent much of Thursday going back through school's self-evaluation form, having promised Moosh that the following day, my birthday would be all hers. Sitting at the kitchen table, I immersed myself in ensuring that I was presenting a true picture of the school's successes, the actions that we had taken and their positive impact, while being careful to honestly identify areas that required further work and the steps that we planned to take. It was a painstaking task.

Moosh took up station at one end of the kitchen table, quietly reading and refusing my offers to make her drinks, content to be nearby and to wait for the carers to arrange lunch and a drink. It was a strange way to be bonded, but nevertheless, there was something reassuring about her proximity.

I so nearly finished.

My birthday dawned, bittersweet: Moosh's last full day in our house, but holding the promise of a family get together for a Chinese meal to remind me that I was, indeed, a year older and to give us all a chance to be together to give Moosh a proper send off. Before breakfast I sat with Moosh while she gave me my card and present and we pretended to mull over what we would order from Ki Ban and then giggled that she would have Singapore noodles, *as always*, and I would have Szechuan chicken and fried rice, *as always*.

Knowing that I had been working since 4:00am, she was happy for me to finish off the self evaluation form by lunchtime and then we would have the afternoon together, before everyone else joined us in the evening.

"Just make sure that you are telling them how hard you all work and how much you care about those children of yours," Moosh advised, before immersing herself in her book.

Keeping to my promise, I was packing away for the week, satisfied that I could do little more to the report, when the phone rang. I skirted behind Moosh's wheelchair to where the phone hung on the side of the big blue cupboard.

It was Shirley calling from school, "I'm so sorry, Mark, I know you're with Mum, and I know how important that is for her and for you, but Elaine is on the other line in your office talking to Ofsted. They are coming next week. Elaine is doing a great job of taking them through the preliminaries, but we're guessing that you will want to be the one who talks to them later."

"Well, isn't that just perfect timing!" I sighed.

The importance of Shirley's message was clearly audible to Moosh, down in her chair, next to me.

As I replaced the receiver, she patted me on the arm, "School. The inspectors. Go do your job; they need you."

Devastated, I repeatedly apologised as I pulled together what I needed.

With utmost calm, she looked me in the eye and said, "You

gave me this week. You'll never know how much that means. Now go. Give my love to everyone. And don't fail to let those inspectors know how brilliant you all are."

Strangely, despite my focus being split and my reserves being stretched, it had been a week to be treasured by both of us: she was so proud watching me do my day job and the time we actually spent together was balm to our fears.

V

Part Five

The Pen Factory
July 2007

36

The Move

What followed was one of my most impressive ever feats of plate spinning: a weekend of trying to ensure that I did right by Moosh, while making sure that school was as ready for inspection as I had been telling myself.

Having all but finished the self-evaluation report before we were so rudely interrupted, I was certain of the positive picture that we would share of our work and success. However, in our school, inspections almost always brought very human flutters and collywobbles: some people have the confidence or phlegmatism to just put their heads down and do what they always do; while a few hear the word 'inspection' and succumb to entirely understandable jitters.

This time, there was a small number of alarms caused by very good teachers inexplicably losing the power to clearly think a lesson through. As a result, much of that Friday afternoon and early evening was devoted to confidence-boosting conversations about how lessons would go, what resources would work best and how to ensure that the children were enabled to be seen at their best.

It being my birthday and, having already planned to have the Chinese take away with Moosh and the family, we determinedly stuck to our arrangement. My brain was not there, but the food was and so was the family. I am certain that my act of being present and enjoying being the centre of attention fooled nobody, but I was happy to feed Moosh her Chinese and blow out the candles on my cake and savour a large glass of merlot, while Moosh sipped just a small whisky and coke, not up to the gleeful guzzling that we had sometimes witnessed in her short time with us.

I have no idea how we fitted it all in, or in what order, but, over the two days of the weekend, we balanced inspection preparation and Moosh moving.

I did not want people slavishly putting in the hours at school, over the weekend, just so that they felt that they had done everything possible, but was grateful that a handful came in for a much needed tidy up. The building was almost derelict and a school fortnight away from being demolished (one week before the summer holiday, and one after), but we tried to put a gloss on the decay. A small group set about hiding junk that was being stock piled for the end of term skip and putting away resources that were scattered around the school due to end of term tiredness. Her Most Wonderfulness came into undertake a single-handed litter pick, convinced that any crisp packet found by the inspectors would be seen as proof of the children being poorly behaved. She still grimaces when she recounts her epic travails of having to wrestle the packets away from vicious, man-eating slugs the size of a guinea pigs.

I tend to be one of those who will keep finding work to do to assure myself that I have left no stone unturned and would, ordinarily, have stayed longer at school, double-double-checking, despite knowing that every sensible step had been taken. This time, however, settling a little, old lady was my priority.

Following Moosh's strict instructions, I asked Fr. Guy to visit our house to perform the Last Rites for her. I had not seen the sacrament given to Moosh by Tank, and it was a little surreal to witness her taking an active, embracing part in the ritual prayers. For me, it was both, on the one hand, distressing that she was clearly aware that her life expectancy was numbered in days or, at most, a very small number of weeks and, on the other, enormously uplifting to see the comfort that she took from receiving absolution and communion.

I knew that these acts made her feel ready to meet God in the hereafter, but, being lulled by the rhythm of the prayers, I was entirely unprepared for Fr. Guy to bring things to an end with a cheery, "There you are, Geraldine: you are good to go."

I was stunned by what I momentarily took to be his inappropriate light-heartedness, until I saw Moosh's beatific smile.

As I saw him out, I expressed very genuine gratitude to Fr. Guy for the succour that he had given to Moosh.

There being nothing left to prevent us, and wanting to have time to recover afterwards, I packed the Zafira in readiness to transport Moosh to her final home. We had agreed, Moosh, Ranjit and I, that it would be just the two of us who went to the home, so the children joined Ranjit to give hugs and kisses and encouragement to Moosh, before she too was packed into the car.

I was expecting a solemn silence on the short drive to the nursing home, but Moosh suggested that I put Westlife on the CD player and we drove through Bearwood with her humming along to 'When You're Looking Like That' blaring from the speakers. That song still brings an enormous grin to my face.

Once we turned into the nursing home car park, I seemed to take an age to park, changing space twice to position the car close to the door. I think that I was more anxiety riven than Moosh. She was the one returning to institutionalised life, to be cared for by strangers, but I was the one abandoning her.

If I could have, at that moment, I would have said, "Look, Ma, we don't have to do this. We can try to find a way of looking after you at home."

Sadly, that was not true and so I quietly asked, "Ready?"

Moosh gave me a small, but enormously brave and determined nod.

We were welcomed at the nursing station by the nurse who had shown Moosh around on our tour, but whose name I had forgotten. As she reintroduced herself as Sylvia, I had no idea that she was about to become enormously important in the lives of Moosh and I.

I knew that we would need to talk through medication and diet. Moosh's current level of need having already been discussed in detail on our previous visit. First, however, Sylvia gently suggested that I spend some time with Moosh in her room, pointing to the one that we had spoken about, in direct line of sight from where we stood at her station, only ten short steps away.

I turned Moosh's chair and wheeled her to her new front door, imagining her holding her hands out to press them against the door frame to prevent us from moving inside, but she didn't, she sat quietly in her chair and then looked around at Sylvia, who had followed us in to speak privately, directly to Moosh.

"Geraldine," she said, "we have given you this room, as we discussed when you visited, because you said that you would prefer to have your meals by yourself. If you decide that you would like to come out to be with some of the other residents for activities, all you need to do is tell one of the girls."

"Thank you, that's kind, but no. I like my own company." Moosh insisted, confirming her previous assertion.

"That's not a problem. I will make sure that the staff understand your wishes and we will make sure to check in on you frequently."

With that, Sylvia left us to take in Moosh's surroundings.

"If you tell me where to put things, I can unpack," I offered.

Attentively, I followed Moosh's quiet instructions to hang blouses, cardigans and jackets and pack away trousers, leggings, vests, pants and socks. She became more positively animated when she asked me to hang her crucifixes. I quickly checked with Sylvia that I was allowed to use the small nails and hooks that I'd brought, and then hung the crosses and photographs of Dad and her mother and one of her with Alex, Arun and Ayesha. She told me which books and magazines she would like near at hand on the wheeled table that rested over the bed. We played around with the position of the television, moving a small chest of drawers to one side of the

271

wardrobe and then back, as Moosh decided which would give her the best vantage point. I folded her wheelchair and stowed it in the corner along with her Zimmer, before we surveyed our joint handiwork.

Using intuition borne of experience, Sylvia reappeared once the bulk of the settling in was done and Moosh accurately talked her through her medication. When Sylvia enquired about her dietary needs, Moosh assured her that there was nothing that she could not eat, but stated that on Fridays, being a Catholic, she would take no meat.

As Sylvia made notes, Moosh pronounced in a mock haughty tone, "I'll eat anything as long as it is tasty."

Sylvia grinned and replied, "A lady who knows her mind. We are going to get on just fine. I'll pop in, once Mark has left, to make sure that everything is as you want it."

"You should go; you need to get ready," Moosh suggested, but I waved her words away.

I was transported back to the moment, over thirty years previously, when, roles reversed, Moosh had been about to leave me in the dormitory on my first day at boarding school. I remembered that, all those years ago, it had been me assuring her that I was ready for her to take her leave.

I knelt next to her chair and enveloped her in the most crushing hug that I dared give her, fearing that she might break or suffocate, until she double-tapped me on the shoulder to tell me to release her, flooding my brain with another childhood memory of play wrestling in which the double-tap signified submission. She smiled, sharing the memory as she brushed my cheek.

I gave the small space a final once-over. The vase of precious flowers cut from Moosh's beloved garden and the array of potted orchids and framed photographs of her grandchildren on the windowsill leant a personalised touch to her new room, providing a sense of homeliness in which to see out the few days that she was believed to have remaining or, more optimistically, a suggestion that she intended to stay for a while.

I left Moosh with faux cheerful promises of returning on Tuesday to find how she was doing and to see if she needed anything and that Ranjit would visit on her afternoon off.

As I left the car park, my head swam with an unspoken, but undeniable recognition that Moosh and I shared: whatever the future held, however brief or long it might be, I had just installed my mother in her final residence.

37

The Great Scrabble Tournament

The first Saturday after Moosh's admission to the nursing home was the first weekend after our inspection.

The two-day inspection had gone well; very well.

By morning breaktime on the Monday, just two and a half hours in, the lead inspector and his team had already judged us to be a good school, so the next day and a half were about as relaxed as it is possible for an inspection to be. This was doubly remarkable, given that the children, staff and inspectors were surrounded by several hundred huge, bright orange packing cases; empty ones in stacks as tall as a short teacher and heavily laden, packed ones, in stacks of three, in any safe space in the classrooms and corridors.

Seeing us in all our semi-packed glory, the lead inspector had asked whether I had considered asking for a dispensation. When I answered that, with my mother on the verge of being transitioned into a nursing home, when the Ofsted call had come, it had never even occurred to me, he reluctantly conceded that such a request would probably have been refused anyway.

He was a very human inspector and was keen that I should visit Moosh at the end of the first day of the inspection (but, having already gauged me, he acknowledged that I probably wouldn't). Once we were completed, his last words to me were to urge me back to the important focus of settling Moosh into her new surroundings.

Had we followed inspection tradition, we would have gone out on the Friday to celebrate our success, but I was relieved to be told that the staff were simply too tired. It was a sad state of affairs, but the holiday was round the corner; we had a school to pack in readiness for our move; we were closing early for the summer to prepare for the full removal of the school to the new building over the next eight weeks; and we were clinging on to any remaining fragments of our collective sanity. We would have drinks in those last couple of child-free days of term - *if* we could find it in us.

I headed to the nursing home with everything that I thought might be useful in helping Moosh to make the most of the time she had remaining (more CDs, an array of magazines and word search puzzle books and industrial quantities of Bournville chocolate).

I was utterly wiped, drained to the marrow, but had prepared myself psychologically to tend to Moosh's needs, in whatever way they presented: changing pads, creaming, dentures, mobile ready for a phone call to Aly, emotional pep talk - you name it, I was mentally ready to be positivity personified.

I arrived and entered, shoulders back and ready for anything, received a warm, smiling nod from Sylvia, at the nursing station, and turned the corner into Moosh's room.

She was sitting up, as perky as I had seen her in over a year, teeth in, neatly presented, washed and groomed and smelling fresh, with even a hint of her favourite perfume. This was my mother who was, now, just a maximum of two weeks from her predicted death.

Trying not to openly gawp, I moved the second chair round so that we could sit at right angles to one another and be close, and I settled myself at her level. Attempting to appear intent on unpacking the goodies from my bags, I surreptitiously inspected Moosh, casting furtive glances in her direction. Reminding me of a small but boldly inquisitive sparrow figuratively hopping from one item to the next as she touched each offering, the appearance of Moosh being vivaciously alive was further enhanced.

Wanting to do nothing more than wallow back, allowing exhaustion to slough over me, I guiltily assessed whether there were any tasks that needed my attention, but everything appeared to be in hand and in very good order. There was an empty bowl on the table, so well emptied that I could not guess what food had been in it.

"What did you have to eat, Ma? Was it good?" I enquired.

"Vegetable soup and bread and butter. It was bland. It needed more pepper," she reported.

"You seem to have polished it off. It can't have been too bland," I observed. "Shall I bring you a secret stash of pepper?"

"Would you? It was OK." she conceded a little begrudgingly.

"How are they looking after you?" I pushed for further concessions to the care that was clearly evident.

276

"They are doing their job well," still grudging, but another acknowledgement from Moosh of the attention that was being paid to her needs.

"Good. That's good." I said, hoping that my relief was not too obvious. "Can you just give me a minute? I need to go ask the nurse a couple of questions."

Moosh shooed me out, grabbing one of the word search books and a pen and I popped out to the nurses' station, pulling the door to, behind me.

I waited while another resident's relative was politely attended to and then quietly asked Sylvia how Moosh had been and was told that she was settling well. She was eating well and her medication regime was in place but would be kept under review. The doctor was due to visit in the next week, so more would be known then. Moosh was interacting well with the staff who were caring for her, but was resisting all invitations to come to meet any of the other residents.

Finally, I came to the crux of what I wanted to say: "She looks fabulous, much better than she has at home. I feel awful that you must be giving her better care than we were able to. Everything seems to have been done. Do I need to change her or do anything for her?"

I will remember the answer I was given to my dying day, because it transformed my life, "Mark, tending to your Mum is our job now. That is what we are here for. It is not uncommon to see an uplift in new residents, as we can care for them round the clock with our staff working on rotation. We will try to do everything for her and, if we don't, you must tell us. If we do that, when you come, you can just love her. That will do her the world of good."

I remember floating back into Moosh's room on an updraft of the deepest gratitude, such was the unburdening effect of that assurance: *when you come, you can just love her*.

Moosh was still engrossed in her word search, so I took full advantage and suggested, "Ma, do you mind if I have a fifteen-minute power nap and then maybe we can play Scrabble. How does that grab you?"

"I was going to suggest that you have a snooze. You do look exhausted. I'm a bit surprised that you came, but I'm very glad you did. Sleep."

She smiled, pushing a bar of Bourneville across the table. I ignored the chocolate and crashed without a second's pause.

Later, possibly more than fifteen-minutes later, I surfaced refreshed and searched out the Scrabble box from the floor of the wardrobe, and, as Moosh watched eagerly, I set out the board and letter holders, score pad and dictionary, bag of letters and a bar of Bourneville.

The box never returned to the bottom of the wardrobe and would stay on Moosh's table for the remainder of her stay, a permanent fixture, for that day we began our Scrabble Tournament.

Such was the excellent quality of care that she received, Moosh would enjoy, not just a fortnight of Scrabble, but close to 500 games over the coming months and years.

When Moosh had lived at her house in Shakespeare Road, I had almost always been rushing back to our house to Ranjit and the children. When I visited Moosh in Loftus, we had managed the odd game, but no more than a handful. In her months at our house, I had promised Moosh innumerable times that we would play more often, but attending to her needs had been my priority. I could stretch to longish conversations, maybe thirty-minutes, which is pretty good going for me, but a game of Scrabble takes time that I rarely found.

Now, here I was being told that my time with Moosh was for me not to tend to her, but to love her, and she loved Scrabble, so it became the thing that we always did. We would read the papers and chat about life, the news, sport, the children, friends, school. We would watch television with *Murder She Wrote* becoming a firm favourite, with a bit of *Columbo* thrown in, but there would be at least one game of Scrabble every week, often two, sometimes three. If I visited on a Tuesday or a Sunday, we would sometimes play five games a week. She never won, not once, and she never cared.

She would cheat, hiding *E*s to be used in an emergency: she *always* needed *E*s. She *hated* *I*s and so she would sneak them (and any other letters that she didn't like the look of) back into the bag and blatantly look in the bag to seek out the letters she wanted. I set myself the target of scoring a minimum of 372 and going 'all out' (using all my letters for a bonus score of 50) in every game. I would bamboozle her with words that I had found in the dictionary – how sad is it that I used to think up words and check them in the dictionary to be deployed at the next opportunity, words like *xi* and *jo* and a raft of words using Q. More than anything, I loved using words which my prudish Moosh would think were rude. Words like my all-time favourite, *yoni*, would utterly scandalise her and she would hoot with bladder endangering glee. We would sometimes spend hours over a game and, if we had to admit defeat, because it was way past bedtime, I would store the board, the bag, and our racks of letters on top of her wardrobe ready to be resumed at the earliest opportunity.

Looking back, there must have been countless other ways, far more constructive ones, for us to pass our time together, but I tell myself that the mental stimulation must have done Moosh good.

What I know, with absolute certainty, is that she took the time that we frittered away on that board game as the token of affection it was intended to be.

And she adored it!

38

Grandchildren And Other Visitors

The window of Moosh's room faced out onto the Bearwood Road, but it could just as well have looked out over the Sahara or the Serengeti, so cut off was she from the community around her.

She could not even see the Bearwood Road, being too short to peer out of the window and too weak to lift herself up high enough to do so.

Moosh held to her declaration made on Day One, that she would not go to eat in the communal area. She didn't want anything to do with the other residents of the home: she effectively isolated herself. Removed from the world, choosing to remain in her room and having lost touch with many of her friends from Church, Moosh saw mainly me and the staff who diligently looked after her.

In the early days, Ranjit was keen to visit her.

She would ask me whether Moosh needed anything bought and would add these to her shopping list. She would always have an eye out for second hand books that she thought Moosh would like, having observed her taste for Maeve Binchy and the like during Moosh's stay with us. She snapped up bargain items of clothing to be added to her package of goods to be taken, always adding little treats that she knew Moosh enjoyed, like dark chocolate *Bounty* bars. She would visit on her afternoons off, rather than join me, arguing that this would increase Moosh's quota of visits. Ranjit was also incredibly good at talking with the staff to monitor how Moosh was and how well she was being looked after, whereas I would just accept that everything was as well as it could be, unless I was informed otherwise.

My blood boiled when I came home to find the wind taken out of Ranjit's sails, because Moosh had made it clear that it was me she wanted to see. At the home, at best, she behaved as if she believed that Ranjit was only visiting out of a sense of duty and at worst, she treated her like a skivvy to be commanded. Undeterred, Ranjit persisted, building herself up for each visit, only to be knocked back each time. She could not hide her hurt, but utterly forbad me from taking Moosh to task over the upset she was causing.

On one occasion, Ranjit took a friend as an ally. The friend reported to me that Moosh had been utterly charming towards her and was clearly delighted to see her, but that Ranjit had almost been dismissed. I already entirely trusted Ranjit's wounded recounts, but hearing them restated by another magnified the pain.

She confirmed Ranjit's view that Moosh's default setting was, "When is Alistair coming?"

Eventually, I told Ranjit not to visit. Although she partially ignored me, the frequency of her visits reduced, which hurt less.

Other friends visited on occasion: Teresa, who had been our friend since college days and who fitted Moosh's "perfect girlfriend" criteria, being "a good Catholic girl" and she having an Irish surname to boot; Sally, our next door neighbour, ten years older than us and a devout Anglican, who seemed to be able to reach Moosh from a caring, faith background. Moosh welcomed both delightedly.

The friends who Moosh especially loved to see were my old school pals, Fred and Dominic. I would never tell her that they were visiting. I would just take them to the nursing home and send them through Moosh's door in front of me. The raucous hoot of delight was a clear indication of her long dormant pheromones being reignited and the flirtation (on her part) was embarrassing to witness, but it was all in good fun.

By anybody's measure, Dominic is, by a very considerable distance, the most badly behaved of all of my friends; he is potty-mouthed and willing to cast a slur at almost anything or anyone if it helps him to get a laugh. If I tried to utter even one of Dominic's most tame *bon mots*, in front of her, I would have been withered in an instant, by a reproving look from Moosh. But not Dominic; he was on the lofty plinth of being my oldest friend and could do no wrong, indeed, the further he pushed his outrageousness the more she loved him.

As far as I could tell, Fred was simply lust on legs in Moosh's eyes, with his confident charm and plummy tones wrapped up in the impressive physique of a swaggering First XV centre/Nigerian prince. Since our youth, Fred and I have had the bond of being deeply respectful admirers of one another's mothers: his mother, proudly robed in floor-skimming, bold prints and wearing eye-catching earrings proclaiming her African heritage, always seemed queenlike to me and he made my mother feel regal. Moosh lapped this up.

Above all others, me included, the visitors who made Moosh's eyes shine the most, and who brought out her very best, were her five grandchildren.

In those years in the nursing home, the thing they all had in common was their power to bring light into her room and to draw love from her. In between their visits, she was surrounded by photographs of them and was always keen to hear about their lives.

Just as with Aly and I, the grandchildren were, rightly or wrongly, compartmentalised in her psyche. They were all special to her, but each in their very own, different ways.

Like me, Alex has always benefitted from being the first born, even if he was only oldest by two months. He got a head start on absorbing a lot of Moosh's affection at a time when I was throwing myself at my career and was still quite newly married, with Ranjit (in Moosh's eyes) being a usurper in the role of leading woman in my life. Moosh was besotted from her first moment with him and lavished her affection and time on him. In his early years, she had given us that enormous support in caring for him, so that we did not have to pay childcare fees. She was instrumental in his development: capitalising on his fascination with naming everything in the world around him; fuelling his love of

284

reading; and nurturing his precocious talent as a pianist.

Alex took his visiting duties seriously, carefully setting aside time to call in and spend an hour or two with her. Each visit rekindled the bond between him and Moosh. He would move away to university in the time that Moosh was in the nursing home, but always made a few hours to visit every time he returned home. She inflated his artistic ego with her adoration and their bond reflected the huge influence that she had in his early years.

While she loved his visits and would croon about them incessantly, when next I visited, she was particularly enamoured if Alex took a girlfriend to meet her. In her eyes, each girlfriend was "the one" and she would wax lyrical about their virtues.

Liam was a wit from the moment he began to express himself.

He looked as if he knew he was an entertainer, before he could speak. He has always had a knack, rather like Dominic, of getting away with the most outrageous comments. In Moosh's queendom, he was the Court Jester In Chief.

Although Liam saw less of Moosh, as a consequence of Aly and Neil moving away from the Midlands when he was seven, his capacity to light up her world with his infectious humour and his joy in pushing boundaries was limitless. Even as an adult, I would quickly be slapped down, were I to dare to utter one of Liam's less offensive quips; not so for Liam of the silver tongue!

His visits were typified by the room struggling for breath and someone having to retrieve Moosh's teeth from wherever she spat them, as another laugh was forced from her and she gracelessly slid from her chair to the floor, with Liam enquiring, "Are you reet down there, lass?"

His crowning glory in the visit-stakes was the day that he spontaneously coerced his friend Diboll, to drive his newly purchased car from Middlesbrough to Birmingham and then to Smethwick to visit Grandma.

In pre-Satnav/Smartphone days, the two of them found their way, fortuitously, to the Bearwood Road and realised, "Hey, there it is: mint!"

Once inside, Liam, divined that Moosh was literally gagging for a whisky and coke. Being her most willing ally in the breaching of rules, Liam set about keeping Moosh entertained, while Diboll was dispatched with directions to the nearest whisky vendor. The two of them had her willingly inebriated in record time and then sloped off back to the North, exceedingly pleased with themselves.

Liam combined with Alex was possibly the most dangerous cocktail of visitors, particularly for anyone in their presence.

Since childhood they had been one another's ying and yang, Liam the blond haired, blue eyed, milky white genetic opposite to Alex's dark curls, brown eyes and olive skin. So different in appearance that neighbours refused to believe that they were cousins, their bond was their laughter. Despite the separation caused by geographic distance and youthful uselessness at keeping in touch, on the increasingly rare occasions that they were together, the two of them clicked back into their childhood partnership of stupidity, the touch paper was lit and mayhem ensued. In most successful comedy duos one is the fool, the other the foil. With Liam and Alex, they simply complemented one another's witticisms, finished each other's lines and goaded the other to greater and sillier daftness.

One evening, not long after Moosh arrived at the home, Liam and Alex found that they were able to coordinate their visit. It was just the two of them and Moosh. Strangely, for Moosh, given that her *Can Do No Wrong Grandsons* were with her, she remained engrossed in David Attenborough's *Blue Planet*, possibly opting for his erudite tones over the inevitable mickey taking.

They proved the wisdom of her choice by adopting Attenborough's voice to comment on Moosh's behaviour, past and present:

Liam: And here we see the Lesser Spotted Moosh in her most vacant form, almost supine, face glazed, teeth held in place by the slightest clenching of her jaw.

Alex: It is rumoured that an adult female Silverback Grandma can consume three times her body weight in dark chocolate Bounty bars. We believe that this must have a considerable laxative effect. We will observe. From a safe distance.

Liam: The matriarch of the Silverback Grandma troupe, who the crew have named Geraldizzle, quietly observes the fish tank awaiting the first move in a fortnight of the Great Big Orange One (otherwise known as The Plant Pot Fish, rare inhabitant of northern hemisphere hospital aquaria).

They were hugely entertained. Liam especially, because, for once in his life, Alex was told by Moosh that she was very disappointed in his behaviour, while Liam was judged to be above reproach. In Liam's words the two of them were 'giggling like muppets in the corner'.

Moosh told me later how much she had loved their antics and loved seeing the two of them together!

287

Arun found it emotionally challenging to visit.

Possibly because he himself was so healthy and active, he struggled in the face of her frailty.

Moosh accepted this with good grace. Sensing his unease, she made the most of seeing him, when she came to our home. In the interim, she avidly read cuttings from the local newspaper in which his football team's matches were reported, glorying in his goals and fist pumping every time he was Man of the Match. Just as she had done with me, she always asserted that he was capable of anything, despite never once having seen him play: her belief in him was total.

Possibly because of their rarity, each of Arun's visits was treated like The Return Of The Prodigal Son. Like Liam, Arun is a wag, but in Moosh's company he was much more reserved, managing to communicate his love, despite being unable to disguise his discomfort in the confines of the home. For her, it was enough that he had made the effort to show his face and she would wait patiently until the next time, without an ounce of negative judgement or regret.

Harvey was utterly special to Moosh in a way that all the rest of us recognised and accepted.

She embraced his uniqueness, his autism and his take on language. He was the one that she raved about, his needs imbuing him with specialness in the most positive sense of the word; he was the one with most pictures in her room; he was her absolute hero. When she had stayed with Aly, Harv was always the most frequent and welcome visitor to her room, her guardian, checking on her visually and in his sensory way.

In the most part, Harv's needs kept Aly in Loftus, as the

logistics of each trip took careful planning and preparation and each of her visits would be followed by weeks of Harv asking for Grandma. When Aly came, it was often more pragmatic for Harv to stay with Neil or for him to be cared for by some of the battalion of Liam's friends. However, on the occasions that Aly did bring him to see her, Moosh would quietly gaze at him, grinning, while he gently held her hand, rearranged her fringe and stared at her, quizzically, as if he was trying to work out where his wonderful Grandma was, lost inside this fading, little lady.

He always cried in the car on the way home, not just at leaving Moosh, but because he found the nursing home unsettling.

Yeeshy was the only girl, which gave her a specialness all her own.

For a woman who was far more at ease in male company and did not have the easiest of relationships with the other key women in her life, Moosh suspended her prevailing antipathy towards the female of the species and adored Yeesh. It was entirely mutual.

Yeesh would happily chat for hours with Moosh, often more freely than with us. In Moosh, she had a reliably present audience and a ready ear, compared to the well-intentioned (but judgemental) nagging and work-squeezed attention span that was her lot at home.

Yeesh happily shared her friends with Moosh, and her Grandma with them. They would traipse the mile and a half there, after school or in the holidays, take her goodies, have a natter and a gossip and then traipse back.

At some point on their walks to and from school, Yeesh

had become more than just a granddaughter, she had begun to be a young carer. Now, visiting her grandmother, despite her youth, Yeesh, just like Ranjit, became a studiously careful monitor of the care given to Moosh, an astute and sensitive questioner of Moosh's circumstances and assessor of her condition, which often resulted in prompting us, "Do you think . . . ?"

Moosh had a confidence in Yeesh, that Yeesh was yet to develop in herself, stating, "She's an astute one, Yeeshy, and very good with people. I'm so proud of her."

On one of her very weak days, fearing for the millionth time that we would lose her, I took Moosh back to our conversation in the garden outside Sheldon Block and asked, "Ma, have you been happy in your life?"

Without a second thought, she answered, "I have been. Some times have been hard, but many have been joyous, especially the years when I had my grandchildren with me."

Her years with her grandchildren were not only her happiest, but also the ones in which she felt that she had given her most and given the best of herself, been most successful and most appreciated. She knew that she was a greatly loved grandmother.

Her years in Bearwood Nursing Home gave her the gift of extending the time that she had to see them grow, not quite to full adulthood. It added greatly to her life to have the love that she had showered on her grandchildren returned with bells on, fivefold.

39

The Escape Committee

Moosh was never going to be the easiest client for any care home or nursing home.

Her determined independence, combined with an increasing cantankerousness, ensured that she would insist, often acerbically, on doing things for herself, which is, of course, a positive trait - unless it puts you in danger.

If she was questioned about why she was doing something her response was likely to be rapid and caustic.

A greater or lesser proportion of each visit would be devoted to me listening to her list of grievances and checking some with the staff, while rationalising others or demonstrating that they were not true. On occasions, I would have to take up issues with her on behalf of the staff, a favourite being that she would refuse to take her medication from certain carers. The truth was that, despite the fact that Moosh could accept that she was being well cared for, she frequently railed against her incarceration.

Moosh never once ever chastised me for putting her in

a home, but she waged a constant series of battles and minor skirmishes to retain her independence: hiding her medication down the sides of her chair; asserting that food was too hot, too cold, too lumpy, too sloppy, too bland; chiding members of the staff; insisting on taking herself off to the loo when that was at least four fumbling steps too far.

The prickliness that she was capable of directing at the staff was a manifestation of her quiet fury at being imprisoned within and betrayed by her body. Difficulties with swallowing and losing her ability to produce her neat, flowing script were all slights that her body inflicted upon her. Having to be assisted with hygiene by people who she did not know was an abject loss of dignity. The challenge of uttering her thoughts through a non-cooperating mouth, where even the teeth struggled to stay, enraged her; not completing her sentences, when the ideas were visible in her eyes, would bring her to tears. Moosh once told me, in broken segments of thought, that she wished that her eyes could be television screens, so that I could see the messages she was trying to tell me.

Her sense of imprisonment was exacerbated by her continued refusal to integrate with the other residents. She was, though, isolated by choice, always abiding by her decision to eat in her room and occupy herself there. The social separation that she chose, rendered her marooned, a small island that welcomed no visits from other residents, just about tolerating the presence of most of the staff. She was content to wait for the visitors who came to see her and for whatever quota of Scrabble games I could manage in any given week.

Much of her life experience rendered her more able than most people to cope with her version of self-imposed, solitary confinement within the home. She had spent almost all of her childhood in an orphanage, never satisfactorily knowing why she was there. She had been single for fifteen years of adulthood before a marriage that frequently saw her stay at home while her husband was off soldiering or socialising. As a foreign looking woman in army quarters, she always kept herself a little apart, or was made to feel separate. When she finally thought that she was going to claim her husband from the army, he drunkenly accepted a job in Iran, leaving her on a Lincolnshire housing estate where she knew no one. He compounded this six years later by taking a job in Saudi Arabia, this time leaving her on a Shropshire housing estate where she knew no one.

In so many ways, she had lived her life alone, which had allowed her to develop a well of resilience strategies in the face of solitude: pushing back against the pesky rules of the home had, seemingly, become one of these strategies.

Nevertheless, there were days when her petty rule breaking and minor insurrections did not give her a sufficient sense of independence. On those days she would make a break for freedom. One of her greatest frustrations was the fact that her legs could not be relied upon to take her to where she wanted to go, but in her early days at the nursing home, she was not willing to allow this to limit her.

I arrived quite late one evening to drop off some washing and some vests and socks that Ranjit had bought. I was in a rush, because I knew that visitors were discouraged after 8 o'clock and did not want to take liberties, so was speeding down the corridor to Moosh's room, when there she was, just opposite the loo, moving quite spryly. She was dressed in her nightie and dressing gown, which was normal, but she was also wearing shoes instead of slippers and, to top off her ensemble, her favourite scarf.

"Ma, why are you using this loo? Is there a problem with your loo?" I quizzed, before applauding, "You've done well to get this far!"

"Ssssh!" she hissed quietly, her finger to her lips. "I'm getting out!"

"Getting out?" I asked, losing my delight in how well she was walking. "To where?"

"Just out!" she scowled, still *sotto voce*, but full of intent.

"Ma! It is cold outside. You have left your coat behind and you have no socks. Where are you going to go? How far are you going to get?" I fired, full of alarm. "And what are you going to say to get them to open the door?"

Being reminded that you needed to buzz the desk to ask them to let you out, and knowing that her plan was foiled, her strength instantly flagged and she flopped against the wall for support.

Gently, I took both of her hands and coaxed her, "Come on, Hogan, let me take you back to your room and we'll talk."

Hogan's Heroes was one of our family favourite TV programmes, when we lived in Germany, a late 60s/early 70s American comedy about a group of POWs in Stalag 13, a fictional camp, who got up to all manner of espionage and sabotage and were always coming up with plots to help prisoners from other camps to escape.

To be fair to Moosh, she was not the only resident who would make a dash for freedom down that corridor. So many of them were at it that I sometimes pondered whether, like Hogan and his buddies, they were co-ordinating their missions. I would frequently meet them, either on foot, in their wheel chairs or stuck at the door holding their Zimmer frames, unable to work out whether to hold the frame or try to push the door.

There was one chap, who I saw so regularly, wheezing at the door in his attempt to get outside for a cigarette, that I asked at the desk whether I should let him out.

Being told that I should not, I took to greeting him with, "Not this time, Mr. Wilkes," before scuttling away from his disappointment.

Back in her room, having passed the empty nurse's station, I could not help but be impressed by the fact that Moosh admitted that she had organised herself (had her shoes and scarf ready), watched for a moment when all the staff were called away from the nurse's station, got her shoes on herself and then made her bid for freedom. I refrained from asking whether she had taken extra drugs to boost her strength, not wanting to give her ideas or to trigger an OAP doping scandal.

When I asked about what she had planned for *after* she made good her escape from the home, Moosh insisted that she wasn't getting out and never coming back; she just wanted to be outside, see outside, see something other than her room. I felt awful, because she never asked me to go out and so, beyond coming to our house, I had not thought to take her anywhere else, so I asked where she would like me to take her.

She wanted to see trees and to go to her Church and so, over the coming months, I built these wishes into my plans.

Seeing the joy on her face as I wheeled her through Light-woods Park, with her admiring the horse chestnut trees was a huge reward, but nothing compared to her delight when I collected her on Sunday and took her to Mass at the Oratory.

For many of her years at Shakespeare Road, I had been pretty good about taking her to Mass for Christmas, but, in honesty, I felt that my holy obligations stopped there. However, when I took her to Mass on those few ordinary Sundays, I could just as well have been showing her heaven.

Sometimes, Moosh didn't even need to go Out Out! Mindful of her susceptibility to bouts of stir craziness, I let Sylvia know, and, after that, a lovely young staff member named Sunil would pop her into her wheelchair and take for a spin up and down the corridor with her gleefully making eyes at him and urging him to go faster. Floozy!

When I suggested that I take her for a few lengths of the corridor, she brushed my offer away with, "Oooh no! It just won't be the same as with Sunil!" Double Floozy!

To my mind, her greatest claim to Steve McQueen's *Great Escape* Hero Status in the escapee stakes was one ordinary Saturday just like most others, when we had played Scrabble, read the papers and put the world to rights.

Moosh was in very good humour and we had spent a joyous time giggling, because I was ribbing her about her fancying Sheriff Tupper on *Murder She Wrote*. I left her chuckling and tightly clasping a chunk of melting Bounty, to nip to her private loo, the one that opened off her room.

The scene that met me behind the door was one of abject neglect. There were brown tiles and plaster all over the floor. I was caught between being desperate to use the loo and anger that my little old Mum was being exposed to such atrocious conditions. Taking one mental step at a time, I used the loo while rehearsing my complaint - I had never been cross or dissatisfied with the home before, so this was a first.

Coming out of the bathroom, something made me ask for details from Moosh, "How long have the tiles been off the wall in there, Ma?"

"This morning," she replied.

"What happened?" I probed.

"I dug them off!" she answered proudly.

"What on Earth for? How?" I gasped, flummoxed.

"I'm tunnelling out!" she grinned.

"And I'm paying for the damage?" I demanded.

She was still grinning, "No, use my money!"

I was never asked to pay. I think they quite admired Moosh's feisty spirit.

(Footnote: For absolute authenticity, Steve McQueen's iconic last hurrah in *The Great Escape* was on a Triumph TR6 Trophy, not in a tunnel, but I was never going to put the idea of a motorbike into Moosh's head! In truth, I included Steve, because he was the first actor my six year old self ever saw Moosh making glorious googoo eyes over (at an open air cinema in Cyprus), before I ever understood what 'come to bed eyes' were . . . *Triple Floozy!*)

40

The Soap Thieves

Saturday visits became a fixture of my life with Moosh. She looked forward to them and, although her demeanour was affected by her health, she was almost always in good humour when I arrived. Even if she was asleep, she would surface from her snooze with an anticipatory smile, her teeth jauntily askew.

So, I was taken aback, one Saturday, to be confronted, by a bristling mother ready to pounce.

"They're stealing my soap!" she accused.

Stalling for time, I slowly deposited bags of laundry and Saturday morning essentials and took time to remove and hang my coat.

"Tell me what's happened, Ma?"

Moosh outlined her grievance, indignantly: "My new bar of Pears has gone. It was in my wash bag. It was still in its box, unopened. I finished the other one and now I don't have one. One of *them* took it. They were in here tidying my room."

Moosh had made accusations of rudeness and slack be-haviour before, about nurses at hospital and carers who visited her in our home. She had even complained about rough handling at hospital, never stating that the roughness was intentional or cruel, but more that she felt that some staff needed to learn to be gentler. She had never made a direct charge of a specific wrongdoing.

This time, her anger was throbbing from her in waves, so much so that a part of me was delighted to see her so pulsatingly vibrant. I found myself caught between sharing her indignation and weighing up previous comments. I was all too aware of newspaper articles and television exposés of residents and clients being maltreated by the staff entrusted with their care and was ready to fight Moosh's corner. At school, one of my key roles was to safeguard children's welfare. Now, here I was having my mother making a disclosure, implicitly trusting that I would address the issue.

On the other hand, whilst still coming to terms with living in the home, Moosh begrudgingly admitted that she was being taken good care off, and, while not every member of staff met with her favour, she had previously conceded that she was treated kindly by staff. This positive view, coupled with the accusations made in hospital and at our own home, led me to be a touch cautious about charging to the nursing station to demand a meeting with Mrs. Sandhu, the owner.

Not wanting to offend Moosh, but wanting to be sure of my ground, I asked, "Ma, I will go and talk to Mrs. Sandhu, but would you mind if I have a rootle around, before I go?"

Knowing that I would be more than slightly disgruntled at not having my own word accepted, I tried to placate her with a smiling reference to one of her lifelong habits, "You always used to have safe places for things that you didn't want to lose. Do you have any here?"

That went down like a lead Zeppelin.

"So, you don't trust your mother!" she snapped. "Search all you like!"

Moosh clamped her jaw shut in her characteristic gesture of volcanic fury and sat in icy silence as I ostentatiously ignored her washbag for fear of provoking a full eruption.

There were no bars of soap tucked behind pot plants or picture frames on the window sill; there were none in the supply of stored pull-ups under her bed and there were none in the bundle of shopping bags next to the wardrobe. I braved Moosh's frosty demeanour to look through the stash of photo albums under the chair she silently fumed in, but nothing.

Her hurt eyes followed me to the wardrobe.

I marvelled at the orderliness of her closet, everything hung neatly or carefully folded. This was so her. She loved order and her organisation made scanning the contents simple. There was nothing on the shelves, the floor or above the cupboard.

However, Moosh had always been a hider. Whether that stemmed back to a childhood in an orphanage, or the life of an army wife trying to squirrel away the housekeeping money from a husband, who, she asserted, would search for it before a drinks night, she had always had boxes and jars and socks, sometimes in plain sight, in which goodies could be kept.

So I frisked her clothes, with her eyes boring into my back, which was how I came to the hard bulge in the pocket of her red jacket: the slightly battered, but unopened packet of a new bar of Pears soap.

Turning, with my hand extended, I showed her the box.

"Ma, that was a particularly good safe place," I said with as much gentleness as I could muster, silently allowing my anxiety to dissipate.

As each step of my search drew a blank, I had been trying to control my anger at the thought of Moosh having her belongings tampered with, while framing my complaint to the management. I had been a few more jackets, all her pairs of shoes and slippers and her washbag away from striding down the corridor to vent my spleen.

Poor Moosh, she looked utterly crestfallen, "I must have put it there to stop it being taken. I completely forgot. I'm so sorry, Alistair."

Her eyes shone with the horror of her error. Blotches of red mottled her tear-streaked cheeks.

Teasingly, in an attempt to relieve our shared tension, I created a small totem pole out of Moosh's teacup, some books and a packet of Arrowroot biscuits, surmounted by the soap box.

"Oh, don't! I nearly accused them myself, but I knew you were coming. Thank goodness I waited."

Her tears continued, despite me shifting from my attempt at levity to simply holding her hands and stroking my thumb over her knobbly knuckles.

"There was no harm done, Ma," I consoled her. "And you let me check, before I confronted the staff, which saved both of our embarrassment."

I waited until her tears subsided, before pushing my luck, "Please be very careful about making accusations. I would hate to be in a position where I wrongly accused a member of staff."

Over the coming years there would be further alarums of the predations of *The Pears Poachers*, interspersed by sporadic spates of *The Bounty Burglars* snaffling Moosh's favourite treats.

Although I took seriously each of Moosh's assertions that her belongings were going missing, I was always careful, with her agreement, to search through potential safe places. Her soaps were either in her jacket or, even more carefully secreted on the shelf in her wardrobe, wrapped in a vest. We never once found missing Bounty bars, because they never made it as far as a safe place. They were kept in front of her on her bed tray, where she could keep a weather eye on them and salivate over them, allowing herself only one minibar on any given day.

Nevertheless, there were visits when she would plaintively tell me that her Bounties were running out faster than they should, due to pesky purloiners. It interested me that she was never as annoyed about the loss of her beloved chocolatey treats, but I would be asked to up her rations to compensate for the toll of the petty thefts.

Months after *The Bounty Burglar* incidents, I was chatting with Sabina, the young woman who had welcomed me on my very first visit. She was regaling me with tales of how lovely Moosh was. Hearteningly, this was not a rose-tinted affection, but included a humorous recognition of Moosh's forthright sharing of opinions and withering chivvying, if she felt one of the girls was slacking, which Sabina acknowledged was sometimes warranted.

What shone through was her sense of the warmth that Moosh could bestow on those she favoured, often demonstrated in the offer of a Bounty bar. It would seem that Moosh was not accounting for her gifting, when she bemoaned the loss of her Bounties. I was greatly encouraged by the idea that Moosh was willing to bring at least some of the staff into the small circle of those that she befriended.

When I quizzed her about her generosity, she positively glowed, which, in that moment, compensated for the difficulty I had in knowing that she was forgetting facts that were important to her. Forgetting where she had put things had the terrible consequence of causing her to feel both violated, at the point of being the victim/accuser, and foolish, when my searches revealed that the things she thought were stolen were either well hidden in one of her crafty caches, or willingly given away.

We always managed to laugh in the end, but, too often, the laughter followed tears.

41

The Birthday Breakout

Moosh would hit the big Eight-Oh in the March after she moved into the home, or at least that is what the calendar optimistically indicated.

Although she was putting up an excellent fight and was having periods of comparative strength and resilience, she was still holding on to life rather than being able to plan for it.

Her End of Life Plan had been set aside, but the hold she had on life was precarious, tenuous at best. Having lived through the summer, when we believed that she had just those few weeks to live, I was hoping that Christmas 2007 was a realistic target for Moosh to live to, but I feared that her eightieth birthday the following March looked overambitious.

I wanted to make sure that she had an Eight-Oh Birthday Party.

One of the joys of our life, at that time, was Sunday nights at

Atticus.

Atticus was a jewel in the Bearwood social scene, a continental-style bar serving well-made food and everything to drink from coffees and teas to imported beers, and offering a vibrant calendar of entertainment.

On Sunday nights it was home to Acoustic Brew's open mic session. A friend had suggested that Alex go down one Sunday night to play, to give him experience of performing in front of a new audience, made up primarily of other musicians and their friends. The first gig had gone well and so there were frequent opportunities to play, either scheduled, or, with us living just a few streets away, Alex would get a call to fill a slot that had become vacant.

We had always enjoyed watching Alex play and became *Atticus Groupies*, if you can be a groupie in your forties. Sunday nights would see us foregoing the traditional teacher end to the weekend of sitting resentfully watching a drama on TV, before trudging to bed and checking the alarm. On the Sundays that Alex was playing, we would call round our friends, and a group of us ranging from teens to fifty-somethings would mosey down to Atticus to watch the acts and listen and applaud, until way past our bedtimes. I maintain to this day that the bands and artists that Alex shared floor space with, while playing for Acoustic Brew, were some of my favourite performers, even compared to well-known, major acts. We were an appreciative audience. A couple of pints of (always lush) Aspall Cyder with friends, and chats with musicians who were, to a fault, wonderfully supportive of one another, was a lovely way to set ourselves up for the week ahead in school.

Moosh vied for the status of Alex's biggest fan, a position for which, modesty aside, there was some competition. She claimed that, as the person who had nurtured his piano playing as a toddler, she was automatically and forever in pole position in the fan club.

At Atticus, I would take photographs and record videos of Alex and other acts, which I would share with Moosh. She would watch them on repeat, utterly rapt. Frequently, she would wrestle my phone away from me, when I tried to retrieve it, so that she could replay a song for the umpteenth time; me wanting to take or make a call meant nothing in comparison to her adoration of her mentee. She did not simply watch to adore, she marked his progress, astutely commenting on his development as a musician and a songwriter. As well as watching video clips, she loved to listen to songs that Alex had burnt to CD for her, covers as well as his own compositions. I would frequently put one of his CDs on for her to listen to, as I was about to leave.

She had loved being part of Alex's eighteenth birthday night, watching him play with his band. Despite her gratitude to us for making sure that she could join us at The Bear, every now and then she would drop into conversation that she had missed part of Knock Door Run's second set through having to get home for bedtime. My teasing reminders that she favoured Westlife over Knock Door Run's punk metal were wafted away.

Alex's sidekick at that time was Diddy, a loveable, hairy, talented drummer.

One night, as Alex and I were dropping Diddy home, the three of us hatched a plan. We would arrange a gig just for

Moosh, for her birthday. We would move the party forward to give her a better chance of living long enough to be part of it. (On the quiet, I told myself that, if she did not survive long enough, the gig would be a fitting send off, a musical wake.) Alex and Diddy would invite other artists to be part of the night and would clear it with Dale and Sam, who ran Acoustic Brew, checking that they would be happy for us to commandeer one of their Sunday nights.

Being a bar, Atticus was a venue open to the public, but Alex and Diddy urged me to speak with Rob about our plan.

When I did, Rob was an absolute diamond, saying, "You choose a Sunday, any Sunday, and we will make it a private function. We can fit eighty people in, so it should be a great night."

For Rob, the fact that it was very good business to have Atticus rammed with happy revellers came a very pale second to the mission of giving Moosh a fitting party. We discussed wheelchair access through the door and creating enough space to ensure that, as guest of honour, her chair would command the best view.

The home loved the idea. Even though I was anxious about telling Moosh about our plans, I wanted to clear the idea with the staff. If they were not supportive, I was prepared to break her out, but their view was that all life enhancing activities were to be encouraged and they were keen to help. I suggested clothes that would be suitable for an eighty-year-old's attendance at a gig and they promised to have her dressed and ready for me to collect.

It was one of the most serendipitous of nights.

Two young lads, a group of their willing muso mates, a

collection of friends from far and wide, a fabulous little venue run by a lovely guy, wonderful support from her carers and a little old lady who just would not give in, all coming together to have a right hooley.

Local friends joined us, our adult friends and the younger set of friends that came with our children. Aly and Neil drove down from the North. Fred came up from London, characteristically arriving late, having been lost on the M42, and therefore raging. (Fred never does anything as mundane as get angry; he moves from Zero to *Incandescent With Rage* at impressive speed, passing the level of anger that most of we mere mortals sometimes achieve in mere nanoseconds.)

Fortunately, the bony embrace that Moosh adoringly bestowed on him, cooled his temper and he stood sentinel over her for much of the night.

The photographs of that party are a carefully archived memento, particularly one of Moosh gazing into the camera, bedecked in a fetching ensemble finished off with a striped scarf in black and several shades of grey (before that ever became a byword for naughty) and a handsome caramel fedora.

Every few years, when I share that photograph on Facebook, Fred posts a message saying, "That's my hat. Mrs. Lanners stole my hat, didn't she?"

The truth is the scarf was stolen too; she liked to steal little bits of those she loved most.

It was an evening of euphoria piled upon delight. The arrival of each new group of guests, heading straight to her to greet her and express affection, care and love, brought Moosh a new rush of pleasure.

In her entire lifetime, I had never seen her be the centre of attention on such a scale, and she was radiant.

In a night of multiple highs, one treasured moment was having her two eldest grandsons sing a duet for her, Liam, in all his dreadlocked glory, and Alex with his impeccably straightened Barnet.

That was only capped by Alex singing 'Paper Plane', a song he had written for her, in which he poured out his fear of losing her and his anger at God. Despite the other eighty people in the audience, he sang to her alone.

And grown men wept.

42

Euro Sex

Another day, another phone call, but this one came on Moosh's birthday, her eightieth . . . the one that I had feared she might not live to see.

Neelam in the office put the call through, "Mark, it's the nursing home. They say that it is important. Can you take the call?"

My heart sank. I was in the middle of having a deeply meaningful conversation with an emotionally challenged nine-year-old, who was having an intensely bad day.

"Give me a moment," I said to Neelam, covering the mouthpiece and directing my attention back to the child, who was still brooding, but gradually calming, "I need you to be very sensible and wait very quietly for me. I need to take this call."

"Yes Sir."

He made himself visibly smaller, hunkering back in the chair.

Taking a breath, I readied myself, "Thanks Neelam, put

them through, please."

"Hello Mark, it's Sylvia. I'm afraid Geraldine has had a fall, this morning. She's hurt her arm.

"We've been observing her and she is in some pain, but not too worried. We think it would be best if she went up to the hospital. We can call an ambulance, but a member of staff will have to go with her and we are a bit short staffed at the moment.

"I know that you are coming later, but I wondered if you could come now. It might speed things up a bit."

I already loved Sylvia, but found myself loving her even more. Her information was always clear, direct and open.

The importance of what was being said, must have translated to my face, because, without hearing a word, my young visitor's own face was showing both interest and concern, before he mouthed to me, "Sir, are you OK?"

I nodded back with a thumbs up.

"OK, Sylvia. Can you give me about 30 minutes. I will take her up to City Hospital. I just need to sort some things out here, first. See you soon."

At the words City Hospital, the boy had sat forward, eyebrows raised and the last signs of his previous bad temper evaporated.

"Hospital, Sir? Is it your Mum?"

He looked at the photo of Moosh and I on top of the aux-speaker on my desk. As a school, we believed that it was important that our children knew that their teachers have real lives away from school and his iffy behaviour ensured that he had visited me often enough over the last few years to know that my mother was unwell.

"Is she OK?" he asked, before adding, crestfallen, "I'm one

of the things you need to sort out, aren't I?"

"It is my, Mum," I confirmed. "She's had a fall and I will need to go to look after her and take her to hospital. And, yes, I do need to make sure that you are OK for the rest of the day. Can you go next door and ask Mrs. Riley whether she is busy, and see if she can come through?"

He positively bounded out of the door like a faithful Andrex Labrador puppy who had found an especially tempting, new loo roll.

Moment's later, he ushered Elaine through my door.

"You need to go," she said. "Your Mum needs you and you need to go take her to hospital. I will look after our young friend. I'll take him now, so that you can pack up."

The lad glowed at the efficiency with which he had reported the level of need, and I grinned at him, "There's clearly no problem with your listening skills, is there? It's a shame that you were having such difficulty concentrating in class. You know you can be much, much better than that, without me nagging you."

"I know, Sir. Mrs. Riley won't need to have me with her. I'll be on my best behaviour. Promise."

He turned to follow Elaine out of the office, but turned at the last minute to pop his head back round the door, "Sir, I hope your Mum will be OK. Good luck at the hospital."

From putting down the phone to reaching Sylvia's station in the nursing home took twenty-six minutes, with no breaking of the speed limit.

Sylvia expanded her earlier message: "She's in good spirits, but I think it is best to get her checked over. She climbed out of bed, over the rails, instead of waiting for the girls to

312

get her up."

When I entered Moosh's room, she looked both sheepish and mischievously triumphant, while making a futile attempt to hide the fact that she was sporting a very conspicuous sling.

"What on Earth have you been up to, this time?" I asked, caught between concern and the twinkle in her eye.

"I was excited. You are taking me out for my birthday!" she beamed. "I wanted to choose something smart to wear. Do you like it?"

She had on a natty combination of black leggings, blue floral blouse, pink socks, sensible brown shoes and her camel jacket draped over her slung arm.

"Very fetching," I conceded. "Have you been flirting with some terrified man?"

"No one." More beaming. "My handsome son is taking me out!"

"Your handsome son is taking you to A&E at City Hospital."

I tried to chide her, but she looked too pleased with herself, so I attempted a glower, "You climbed over the rails and fell all the way to the floor? Not your best escape mission so far, is it? You need to stay safe and wait for help."

"I couldn't wait all day. I can do it myself. Don't be angry with me. It's my birthday. Take me out. Can we still get a Chinese? I'd like -"

"Singapore Noodles? Extra spicy?" I finished her sentence, giving up on the stern face. "Let's get to A&E and see what they can do, first."

Either by good fortune or, much more probably due to Moosh merrily chirping, "It's my birthday. We're going for a Chinese!" to the receptionist, the triage nurse, the young doctor and the x-ray team, we found ourselves in the fracture clinic double-fast.

Nothing had diminished Moosh's enthusiasm; she had flirted her way round the hospital and her mischievousness luminesced round her like a miniature rainbow, even after her treasured jade bangle had to be bolt-cut from her arm and her rings snipped off her swollen fingers.

While the nurse prepared the lengths of plaster to create a pot for her wrist, Moosh leant over to me and stage-whispered, "Do you know that there is a new sex shop in Bearwood?"

The doctor chuckled covertly but the nurse squawked unrestrainedly, "Really, Geraldine? You'll have to tell me where it is!"

I was mortified. My tiny little Just Reached 80 mother, product of a convent upbringing, holier than thou whenever it suited her, with her box full of God words, was here claiming knowledge of a sex shop. In Bearwood. And joking about it!

"Ma! There is no such thing!"

Then, doubting myself and ever so inquisitive, I ventured, "As a 40-something man, living in Bearwood, I think I would have spotted a new sex shop, don't you? Where in Bearwood?"

"I brought you up properly! You're a good boy!" she hooted. "It's down towards Woolies, on the left hand side. It's got a big blue sign saying Euro Sex!"

The doctor was leaving the nurse to fix the plaster cast in place, but as he departed, he called out cheerily, "We'll see you in a few weeks, Geraldine. You've made my night!"

314

"But you've not been to Bearwood, for months," I countered.

"I have! Richard pushes me all the way up there in my wheelchair. I like to see what's happening."

She trumped me with a snippet of successful escapee news that was unbeknownst to me! And who was Richard? Was Richard the Orlando to Sunil's Johnny?

I might have lapsed into a wobble of guilt that it hadn't been me pushing Moosh along the high street, if I hadn't caught the nurse whisper conspiratorially to Moosh, "It's my sister's hen do at the weekend. I'm going to pop up to Bearwood and buy her something naughty! Something with a bit of a buzz!"

Moosh scandalised me, by cackling with delight: she understood *buzz*!

We had just enough time to drive to Quinton to pick up everybody's order, including Moosh's extra spicy Singapore Noodles. I *swear* that the Bearwood Road is on the most direct route from City Hospital to the Chinese *and* that it wasn't wayward curiosity led me to drive that way.

As we approached where Woolies had once stood, Moosh pointed triumphantly, "There! See!"

"*Specs*, Ma! Not *Sex*!" I howled avoiding a mirth-induced swerve into the traffic coming from the crossroads at the Kings Head.

"It says, 'Specs', Ma! And the sign is green, not blue!"

"I wasn't wearing my glasses!" she hoot-howl-cackled, only just managing to keep her teeth in.

Every time I think of that night, I wonder whether the poor

fracture clinic nurse ever came to buy her hen do naughties and stood, utterly confused, looking up and down the high street and then put 2 and 2 together, when she saw the *Specsavers* sign.

Perhaps she grinned at the memory of that little old, young at heart minx, so determined to be out celebrating her 80th birthday.

For myself, even to this day, I have to go to the West Bromwich branch to get my glasses!

43

The Risk Assessment

A direct result of Moosh's spectacular dive from her bed and the resultant arm break was Sylvia politely requesting that we have a talk about the frequency with which Moosh's actions were endangering herself.

Being responsible for risk management at my school, I understood entirely the need to try to put safeguarding measures in place around Moosh, so I readily agreed.

It was not a deeply formal conversation, but it was, nevertheless, a serious one.

Sylvia and the team were concerned that Moosh was continually putting herself in danger. Empathetically, they recognised that Moosh was trying to retain as many vestiges of her independence as she could, but equally they argued that they could keep her much safer, if she would ask for help more often. I fully understood where they were coming from, even down to the hope of cutting down on the paperwork of writing up each incident, necessitated by each of Moosh's accidents.

I knew about the big accidents, because I was called each time they happened. I had been told of a catalogue of smaller incidents. Ranjit and Yeesh almost always had some story to tell when they had visited. I had seen for myself all manner of bruises, cuts and abrasions, all of which Moosh brushed off as hazards of life. Almost all of them had, to some degree, been self-inflicted.

Without doubt, her most spectacular moment was the morning that she pulled the wardrobe door off its hinges and onto herself, causing a new patchwork of bruises. When quizzed about how this had happened, she indignantly informed me that she was choosing her clothes when her legs gave way and she grabbed hold of the nearest thing: the door. She insisted that she should not be blamed for the wardrobe coming apart and that I should take the matter up with Mrs. Sandhu. I did not tell her that, having had to catch the dead weight of her plummeting floorwards, on more than one occasion, my sympathies lay with the wardrobe.

What I was unaware of, prior to my talk with Sylvia, was the full litany of falls, collapses and collisions with static objects, that went beyond her furniture dismantling episode. The incidence was not quite daily, but several accidents were happening each week. The injuries rarely required medical attention, beyond first aid, but what every incident demanded was that a record was made.

Documentation takes time and, in almost any profession, is the bane of employees' lives, taking them away from the job that they thought they were signing up for. I knew that in education, teachers and school leaders felt inundated with all manner of paperwork that takes the joy out of working with children and, while I never managed to fathom the vocation that led a person to choose to work in a nursing home, I could understand that the paperwork caused by Moosh's stubborn insistence on doing things for herself, was causing an unwanted burden.

"How would you like to play this?" I asked Sylvia. "How can I help?"

"Well," she paused, instigating a sudden fear that Moosh was about to be expelled, but I rationalised that, if that were about to happen, there would be a sit-down meeting with the manager.

Sylvia continued, "I was hoping that you would have a chat with Geraldine and convince her to ask one of us for help. We are here to help Geraldine. If she calls for one of us, we can go to her. She can then do what she wants to do, like get her clothes out, or go to the bathroom, and we can be there to help her, hovering, and only stepping in if she needs us. How does that sound?"

As relief flooded through me at the confirmation of the non-expulsion of Moosh, I managed to catch myself before I reached across the counter to kiss Sylvia, such was my gratitude.

Instead, I gushed, "Of course I'll talk to her. I'll go in and see her now. I'll let you know how it goes!"

Without taking time to develop a line of argument, I took the few steps from Sylvia's desk to my chair in Moosh's room.

She twinkled, as I appeared, raising her plaster cast in a proud, rakish salute, with clearly no notion of the workload that her most recent dive had caused, or all of the other accidents that preceded it. She just looked pleased to see me.

"Hi Ma, how's the arm? And how are you?" I opened.

"I can't complain, can I? It was my own fault, but it's OK, actually, not too bad," she said, taking on a slightly abashed hue. "It's nice to see you."

"Aren't you the lucky one?" I quipped, before continuing, "I need to talk to you about something."

"This sounds ominous," she remarked, her rakishness completely evaporated.

"No, not ominous, but there is something I need us to think about," I tried to reassure her. "The thing is, I've been talking to Sylvia about the accidents you've been having and trying to see if there is a way of keeping you safer, so that you don't do yourself even greater damage."

"And?" she began to look affronted.

"And," I went on, "I need you to start to use your button more. When you want to go to the loo or move around your room, I need you to call for help."

Despite sensing her hackles rising, I persisted, "It will save you from getting hurt. It is not about trying to stop you from doing things for yourself. It just means that one of the staff will be here to help you, if you need them. They will not interfere, unless you are in danger."

I was quietly pleased with myself that, without planning my spiel, I had instinctively omitted words like *monitor* and *supervise*, *assist* or *risk* or any other of my manager speak, but seeing the onset of her truly annoyed cat's-bottom-mouth and visible puffing up from her usual miniature size, I played my ace.

"If you won't ask for help, there is a good chance that they will refuse to have you here, and you know that we can't have you at home, so we'd all be more stuffed than a Christmas turkey."

With determined satisfaction, I saw that her balloon was well and truly burst, withering from the mildly terrifying, Zeppelinesque warlike volume of a moment earlier. Instead, she looked tired and deflatedly limp.

"If that is what you want," she conceded.

In my brain I chanted my success mantra, "He shoots! He scores!"

And then, completely mixing my competitions: "Check mate!"

I consoled Moosh with a couple of morale boosting games of Scrabble, purposefully not scoring any seven-letter words and keeping my scores to the low 400s.

Before I left, I promised her, "We are all only trying to keep you safe. We like having you around."

She looked fully appeased and offered her own promise, "I will behave. I'm not trying to make extra work for anyone. I like to do things for myself, but I will make sure that I am patient."

As I drove away, I congratulated myself on my stunning strategy and the resulting victory.

Stupid me!

On Saturday, I arrived in Moosh's room to find her perched expectantly on her chair.

She was clearly waiting for me. In her hand, which was resting on her lap, was a little leather-bound book that I had noticed before, without ever properly registering it. It was usually on the trolley-table that could be wheeled into place over her legs, so that it was in front of her when she sat up in bed.

Before I could even greet her, or put down my bags of the

usual Saturday morning essentials, Moosh thrust the small book at me saying, "I'd like you to read something."

I noted that a bookmark had been put in place, which allowed her to quickly move to the page she wanted, and I saw that she had drawn a series of lines around a sizeable section of text; she was never shy about defacing books.

"Please read the part that I've highlighted," she requested with signal determination.

I have tried to locate that passage in the intervening years, but try as I might, my attempts have been without success. I can, however, remember the gist very clearly. What I can visualise even more vividly, is the look of vindication that I saw blooming on her face, as I looked up after each silently read sentence. The text was a Christian one in which the reader was exhorted to use all of the faculties that had been bestowed upon them by God and warning that not to do so was to dishonour Him.

"You see, Alistair," Moosh said, without the slightest hint of triumph, "while I can get up and walk and do things for myself, I must. If I don't, then I am wasting the gifts that God has given to me. While I have the strength to be independent, I must."

I had absolutely no riposte, not one.

Instead, I asked, "So what do we do now?"

"Well, I was thinking that if you talk to Edith and explain, maybe she will understand," Moosh suggested. "I know that she is a Christian and her faith is important to her. I think she will know what I mean."

A part of me was delighted and impressed by Moosh's own strategising and carefully calculated preparation.

"Shall I go find her now?" I asked.

"Would you?" she asked.

Edith was the manager of the nursing home.

Armed with Moosh's little book and the marked text, I knocked on Edith's door and was greeted in her richly, mellifluous, southern African tones. I explained that Moosh had asked me to show her a passage from the book and that Moosh believed that it would help people to see why she was trying to do things for herself.

Without question, Edith read in silence and then looked at me, her eyes misting, "She's right. She's a devout Christian lady and this is important to her. I will explain to the girls and we will monitor her every 15 minutes and ask her, each time, if she needs anything."

Edith walked back down to Moosh's room with me and I showed her in. She went straight to Moosh, knelt down next to her and embraced her with great warmth and tenderness and then spoke to her in a voice that conveyed shared devout belief.

"Geraldine, you are an example to us all. We sometimes forget ourselves. You keep honouring God and we will keep looking after you."

The look of gratitude on Moosh's face melted me.

Just like all truly great champions, Moosh never rubbed it in, but it was one of her greatest victories, certainly one that was hugely important to her: she had the go ahead to maintain her precarious independence.

44

The Malayans In The House

On the first Saturday after the summer holidays, I was making a planned pit stop around the corner from the nursing home.

The newsagent off the roundabout at the end of Cheshire Road had become my provision store of choice, as it always stocked both Arrowroot biscuits, and Nice, which were now on Moosh's Saturday morning shopping list. Standing in front of a stack of boxes of Tunnock's Chocolate Teacakes, I was tracking back through my early life memories to consider whether these were something that Moosh might like to have added to the hamper of biscuits and chocolates of my childhood that I bought for her each week.

As I was lost in pondering a silly game with those teacakes (a game that I only half remembered, thinking that it was something we had played together in my childhood), I realised that my mobile phone was ringing.

Seeing Ranjit's name on my screen, I answered, "Hi there, I didn't forget anything did I?"

My brain was still niggling at the teacake game.

"Mark," the slightly panicked tone that Ranjit managed to imbue my name with, snapped my mind away from a glimmer of chocolate and marshmallowy meringue stuck to a forehead, even before she squawked, "there are two Malayan people standing in our living room!"

To this day I still giggle to myself that, if Ranjit had said *Martian* instead of Malayan, I'm certain that she could not have sounded more flustered.

Then she added, "And they are looking for Geraldine!"

Entertaining visions of tiny aliens arriving from Mars and demanding to see Geraldine, the leader of this planet, had me whispering back, "So, if they are in the living room, where are you?"

"In the kitchen!" she hissed.

"How do you know they are Malayan? Did they come all the way from there, today, to stand in our living room?" (I was enjoying this.)

"No! They came from Hilltop!"

"Is that part of Malaya? Near Kuala Lumpur?" I asked innocently.

"No! It's past West Brom. Stop teasing me! Please can you come home. They asked to speak to Alistair. Sandra sent them."

Sandra is my aunt, my mother's youngest sister. My interest was piqued.

"Let me just pay for my shopping and I'll come home," I promised, adding the teacakes to my basket.

On the five-minute drive home, I pictured Sandra.

I had last seen her when I was at teacher training college.

I had been summoned home to meet my ailing grandfather for the first and last time in my life. He had flown from Malaya with Sandra and my young cousin, Sasha. They had visited London to stay with Sita, an aunt I had never heard of until that visit, and bring her to Shropshire to stay. Grandfather was very ill, suffering from diabetes and had had one leg amputated. I knew about his illness, because Moosh had been in touch with him for several years and had told me about the repeated amputations to try to remove the gangrene in his toe, then his foot and finally his leg. I remembered Sandra as his exotic carer and protector and organiser of the trip: warm, friendly, kind, a real doer and life force.

That is all I had.

In those days, I angrily associated Malaya with my mother's childhood, abandoned in the convent orphanage, and I must confess to keeping myself rather aloof from the family reunion.

What I did remember clearly, however, was that Moosh was very fond of Sandra.

Arriving home, I did indeed find two Malayans in the living room, although by now Ranjit had calmed down and offered them drinks and they had been invited to sit. I had visions of finding them still standing. They did not look even vaguely like Martians, nor scary.

"Hi, I'm Alistair. Well, I'm Mark, but people that my Mum knows call me Alistair," I introduced myself, shaking hands.

"Ranjit told me that Sandra sent you? My auntie Sandra? From Malaya?"

What followed was a heart-warming tale of sisterly devotion as the woman, Bally, explained, "We have known Sandra for several years now. She has been trying to make contact with her sister, Geraldine, your mother.

"She has your mother's address at Shakespeare Road and has stayed with her there, before, but she has been unable to contact her by phone.

"She asked for my help, because she knew that I could access data through my job. Please don't tell anyone, because I could get into trouble, but I accessed the data base at work and searched for addresses linked to your name. I could not find an A. Lanyon, but we decided to gamble on M. Lanyon, which is how we found you.

"I think we alarmed your wife. We're terribly sorry. We did not mean to."

Ranjit looked mortified, "No, please, I was wrong-footed. Your visit came so out of the blue, but I'm so pleased that you have come. It fills a huge gap. Geraldine will be ecstatic."

Bally produced a sheet of paper, "I have your aunt's contact details, which she asked us to give you. Please would you email her to let her know that we have found you. I have added our details. Please let us know how you get on."

What I had taken for panic in Ranjit was, in fact, effervescing excitement that she was struggling to contain.

"Isn't it fantastic!" she exclaimed, tears in her eyes and chin quivering, after Balraj and Bally drove away.

"They've made such an effort to track you down. We can have Sandra and Geraldine back in touch. Take Sandra's phone number to your Mum. She will be over the moon."

I, too, was euphoric. Just knowing that Moosh mattered to someone, beyond the close group who had been supporting us for the last few years, was fabulous. To know that her importance had triggered a real-life womanhunt (and some well-intentioned rule breaking) made it even more wonderful. I was certain that Moosh would be overjoyed.

However, before I built up Moosh's excitement with the prospect of a phone call to her sister, I wanted to gauge Sandra's position, so I told Ranjit, "I'm going to email Sandra and see how she wants to play things. I will just tell Mum that Sandra has been in touch."

As I completed my earlier journey, I did consider for almost an entire millisecond whether the news might overwhelm Moosh. That decided, I managed to prevent myself from rushing headlong into her room.

I remained calm for long enough to dole out some Arrowroot and Nice and settle into my chair before announcing, "Moosh! Auntie Sandra's been in touch. She's been trying to find you and, when she could not, she asked her friends to search for you. They came to our house this morning. They were lovely. And I have her email address!"

My words tumbled out, a small torrent of my own excitement.

"I have her email, here!" I repeated, waving the slip of paper. "What would you like me to say to her for you?"

While I jabbered, Moosh's eyes had grown to fill the portion of her face that was not taken up by an enormous grin. Otherwise she was perfectly motionless, her normally writhing body stilled. She glowed.

"She's been searching for me? I prayed that I would see her one more time."

Her eyes glistened and a tear escaped, but she continued

to grin.

"Yes, let's email her. I want you to tell her that I love her, and I miss her, and I'm so grateful that she has made the effort to find me. How do I email her? I've never sent an email!"

"Don't you worry, I'll send her all of what you've just said in an email, and she will get it straight away, or as soon as she looks at her emails." I smiled.

"What? She'll get it today?" she beamed. "That's rapid! So, I could hear back from her today?"

All of the excitement was too much for both of us and we both fell asleep.

I dread to think what the happy snoring sounded like.

On Sunday evening, I returned, with Sandra's emailed reply.

I had made certain that I had sufficient charge on my phone.

I am certain that I was at my most unabashedly Tiggerish, as I bounced into Moosh's room, waving my phone and declaring, "They are eight hours ahead in Malaya, aren't they? It's 2:30am there, but Auntie Sandra says that she stays up late. Come on, we're going to ring her!"

To be fair to her, Moosh took this announcement in her stride, with far more calm than I could muster, as if she had been patiently expecting that God would allow her one more contact with her sister.

I keyed in the number, placed the handset in her hand and pressed dial.

As her illness progressed and her condition deteriorated, mobile phones had become Moosh's enemy. She could never get them the right way round, or the right way up, and she was forever inadvertently terminating conversations. None of that happened.

She held the phone confidently, waiting for the connection, before squealing, the calm facade entirely gone, "Sis! It's me!"

I had witnessed this once before.

Nine years earlier, I had fulfilled a promise to Moosh that I would track down her elder sister, Marguerite, in Australia. With nothing to go on other than her name and a country, a friend had fortuitously suggested that I search the Australian white pages on the internet. We searched city by city and, aided by a unique hyphenated surname, came up with precisely one match in a continent of over 19,650,000 souls. The odds were, literally, lottery level. The number got me through to the ex-wife of one of Marguerite's sons, Charlie, and within hours I had Moosh talking to Marguerite after an interval of forty-seven years, and me talking to my cousin, Ann.

Moosh's delight in that conversation with Marguerite was matched by the unbridled joy of her reconnection with Sandra. As is so often the case with friends who have lost touch for long periods, they took up where they had left off.

In 2002 Moosh had got on a plane at the age of 74 to travel across the world to hug the older sister that she had thought she would die without ever seeing again. In 2009, she and her younger sister joyously hatched plans to replicate the mission. This time Moosh could no longer travel, so Sandra would.

To celebrate I taught Moosh the teacake game - it wasn't one of our family games after all; it came from our friend Annabel.

You unwrap the teacake from its red and silver foil wrapper, place it on the palm of your hand and smack it on your forehead. You have to use just the right amount of smack to crack the chocolate shell and reveal the gooey white centre, but, without getting even the tiniest smidgen of luscious marshmallow on your skin.

Moosh loved it! (If you haven't ever tried it, *do*!)

For most of us, the act of striking our forehead with our hand is something we take for granted, but the difficulty that Moosh had in controlling her limbs meant that a few teacakes flew around the room and had to be binned. She squirmed with laughter at the sight of me coated in splodges of marshmallow and shards of chocolate, after I intentionally smashed my second teacake right in the centre of my forehead. She then put every ounce of concentration and body control into smashing her own white and brown Cyclops eye.

We were crying blissfully and gasping for air.

The look on the faces of the two young carers, drawn by our peals of laughter and peeking into the room, was an absolute joy.

Moosh and I were high on teacake and the anticipation of Sandra's visit.

45

The Airport And The Inspector

What followed was one of those whirlwind fortnights.

The flurry of communication with Auntie Sandra, through emails and phone calls and then Facebook, was exhilarating, not only for Moosh but for Ranjit and me.

By the end of Sunday night, plans were in place for Sandra to visit within little over a week. I have to admit to being mightily impressed that my aunt could reconnect with her sister one week and travel around the globe the next. Sandra assured me that she was not a jetsetter, but that she had already arranged to visit a friend in Germany and, hearing of her contact with Moosh, her husband had suggested that she simply extend the trip, it being silly to come to Europe without taking the extra small step.

In my communication with Sandra, I had been open about the level of Moosh's strength/weakness and, while not quite saying, "She's dying: come now!" I did pounce on the extension to her trip, because I knew that it would lift Moosh in a manner that I never could: Moosh knew that it only took five-minutes to get to her from our house, which pales in comparison to the continent hopping that Sandra had put in motion.

The impending visit brought on the usual bustle of crisis cleaning and tidying to make sure that the office, which doubled as our spare room, was up to standard for our esteemed, world travelling guest, or at the very least not a potential source of contagion. I am blessed with living with three of the untidiest humans in existence, and my office was a favourite dumping ground for unwanted *anythings*, so, I cursed and stomped around, decluttering, tidying, hoovering and dusting in the office, until my embarrassment ebbed, my grumbling leaving everyone in no doubt that certain death would be inflicted on the person who undid my hard work.

At school, we were in a good place.

Our attainment data and our progress data were secure and, more importantly for me, the school felt good: the children were beamingly happy and felt safe; the parents were almost all pleased with their children's experiences in school and felt that they were part of their children's learning, and our staff knew that they were doing a commendable job. We knew what elements we needed to keep building, and there was a strong sense of shared purpose.

We were in that honeymoon period that we generally had at the start of each year. The children were settling in, finding their feet and almost all trying to impress their new teachers, and the teachers and teaching assistants were consistently communicating positive expectations, so behaviour was good, and school felt lovely. We were at least twelve months way from inspection, so were looking forward to a year of providing enjoyable learning opportunities, free from external scrutiny.

When the call came from the inspectorate's administrative team, I actually said, out loud, down the phone, "I think you may have the wrong school. We aren't expecting to be inspected until next summer at the earliest."

The very young man at the other end of the phone said, "Yes, I'm sorry about that, but that's exactly why we are including some schools like yours, to catch you out. The guidance says, 'In the third year after your last inspection', and you are now in your third year. Your inspection will be next Tuesday and Wednesday."

I was quietly fuming that the inspection was plum in the middle of Sandra's visit.

That aside, I was stunned by what I took to be the unfairness of the timing, a feeling that magnified as I juggled numbers with remarkable rapidity, given the pressurised context, and then had to keep a tight grip of my professional demeanour as I asserted, "I appreciate the cunning plan, but an interval of two years and eleven working days since our last inspection does not seem to be reasonable. We don't even have all of our Reception children started yet!"

Reciprocating my professionalism admirably, the young man answered, "I can understand that, and I will make a note of your views, if you would like me to. The lead inspector will call you this afternoon."

I am proud to say that our response as a school was lightning quick, from the meeting with the staff at lunchtime, preceded by the tannoy announcement that school staff live in dread of, "Could all staff please meet in the staffroom at 12:45pm."

That announcement almost always means, "We are about to be inspected!"

We did many of the things that you are not supposed to: staff worked late on Friday and came in on Saturday and Sunday; we abandoned the training session on Monday to allow staff to fine tune their lesson prep and their classrooms; we made sure that *T*s were crossed and *I*s dotted. Not having expected to be inspected, and it being less than a fortnight into the term, I had not read the shiny, new, two-week-old inspection handbook, but I had gathered all of our progress data onto one sheet of paper, and I knew it was good.

We were ready for Tuesday.

Sandra was flying into East Midlands airport at midnight on Monday.

I had made sure that the lead inspector knew this by mentioning it several times.

Ranjit and I drove over to Nottingham at a time of night that I would normally be sound asleep, on a school day. I was so out on my feet, as I waited at the arrivals gate looking for the lady from the Facebook photographs, that Ranjit had to tap me on my shoulder to show me that Sandra had walked past me and was now standing expectantly next to her.

I was delighted to see Sandra again and could not wait to reunite her with Moosh, but the inspection would start in eight hours.

We drove home.

We may have chatted in the car, but I do not remember.

I met with the lead inspector at 7:45am, having arrived at Stupid O'Clock.

She rearranged my office to her liking, as we had nowhere else in school for the inspection team to be based.

The inspectors met the staff at 8:30am and by 9:00am I had shared our data. From the look on the inspectors' faces, as they looked at my proudly proffered single sheet of colour-coded attainment and progress figures, I knew the outcome was going to be positive and, with only a few minor hitches, it was.

The lead inspector applauded the fact that I had 'got on with real life' by collecting my aunt the night before, and made absolutely no allowances for my fatigue. As it turned out, I did not need her to: staff, children, parents and governors pulled together to secure the good judgement that we expected, and the initial feedback was given a pleasing extra lustre by the inclusion of cherished words like *outstanding* and *exceptional*.

Sandra was a fabulous house guest: she cooked mutton curry with crumpets for us; she made a fuss of the children; she went off exploring Birmingham and on a day trip to Stratford upon Avon; she filled us in on the story of how Bally and Balraj found us; and, of course, she visited Moosh.

As both Sandra and I hoped, seeing her beloved sibling revitalised Moosh. For me, seeing these two sisters, who had spent so much of their lives on different continents and separated by life circumstances, finally in the same place, was a privilege that I treasure.

From the first moment, it was bitter-sweet, as we all knew that those few days would be the last time that they would see one another. Each of them treated the hours they spent together as indescribably precious and, while tears fell in abundance, the ardent warmth of their screeches of laughter quickly dried them.

For much of their time together that week, I left them to their sisterly bonding and reminiscing, but after the inspection was completed and before Sandra flew home, we all wanted to take up Bally and Balraj on their invitation to visit them. I wanted to hear more about the finding of Moosh and the three of them, Sandra, Bally and Balraj, were happy to take turns to tell their parts of the story.

Moosh and my aunt, Sandra, are half-sisters through their father. Sandra's own mother passed away in March 1998. Not long after, Sandra suffered a fall in her garden, badly hurting her leg. Feeling entirely low, Sandra decided that a trip to the United Kingdom would help raise her spirits.

Once here, she made her way to Birmingham New Street, but, although she had her sister's address as Shakespeare Road, Oldbury, she did not have the house number. Desperately, or ingeniously, Sandra reasoned that, if she approached the authorities of the cemetery where my Dad was buried, she may be able to find details of his address, but, there being two cemeteries, she had to decide where to start.

Seeing a bus to Smethwick, she boarded, not knowing that she would need the exact change.

As she puts it, "The bus driver was a very kindly person," and he stopped the bus to allow her to go upstairs to ask for change, which she did.

When he asked where she wanted to go, she explained her predicament and he suggested that the best place on his route for him to drop her was the Council House, where, hopefully, someone might be able to help.

Upon hearing her predicament, the woman at the Council

House reception pointed to a man behind my aunt saying, "This gentleman may be able to help you."

The tall, clearly Asian man's first words were, "How may I help you? You're Malaysian? Apa khabar?"

My aunt was utterly taken aback at hearing a familiar language in a foreign land. The gentleman was Balraj, formerly from Malaysia.

Balraj took Sandra to his office, sat her down and started to search for Geraldine on the computer, but had no success.

Concerned, he asked Sandra whether she was sure that her sister was still alive, at which she burst into tears causing him to attempt to placate her with, "Let me look through, once more. Please don't get upset."

At that moment his wife, Bally, walked in and was told the story.

Her solution was simple, "Let's go to Shakespeare Road."

When Balraj asserted that this was crazy, her response was, "I'm a social worker, that's what I do: knock on people's doors!"

Arriving together at Shakespeare Road, Sandra had two guesses.

Receiving no response at either, they decided that Sandra should look through the letter boxes, which is how she spied Moosh's porcelain cats and said, "I'm sure this is the place."

A neighbour informed Sandra and Bally that Moosh was away babysitting, and so they pushed a note through the letter box, and Bally invited Sandra to stay with them.

Two days later, Moosh phoned Sandra at Bally and Balraj's, saying that she had returned and to invite her to stay.

Balraj was concerned about the reception that Sandra would receive from her sister and refused to allow her to take her luggage, so when Sandra arrived at Moosh's, her first words were, "Where are your bags?"

Balraj and Bally brought them over.

Sandra shared that, at first Moosh was not very talkative, but after an hour she was back to the 'normal' that Sandra remembered from years before, with her high-pitched cackle, and so she stayed and they enjoyed three days together, before Moosh had to head off to further babysitting duties.

They travelled together to Stratford upon Avon, so we surmised that Moosh must have been on her way to Aly and Neil's in Leyton Buzzard. Sandra's parting gift to Moosh was a gold bracelet that Sandra had been given by her mother.

When, some years later, Sandra's phone calls had ceased to be answered, she asked Balraj to find out what had happened to her sister. Balraj discovered that Moosh had been hospitalised following a fall, and that her house was being looked after by someone called Mark. Sandra knew me as Alistair, but asked Balraj to trace me.

And as Sandra summarised: "Well, the rest is history!"

I was staggered that I had never known about Sandra's previous visit, but Ranjit rationalised that Moosh's institutionalised, early life experience was often at the root of behaviours, which we perceived were divisive within the family: she rarely ever saw Aly and I at the same time, never once having us simultaneously in her house on Shakespeare Road. I could not understand why Moosh never asked me to contact Sandra or how Moosh was so difficult for Bally and Balraj to find through the records.

Ultimately, none of that mattered: they were together, sharing time as sisters. I could take no credit for it, apart from the airport run. Together, we marvelled at the string of happy circumstances that brought us to Bally and Balraj's house: the kindly bus driver, the fact that Balraj was standing next to Sandra at the council house, the Malaysian connection, Bally and Balraj's generosity of time and friendship.

Moosh *loved* that she had been at the centre of so many people's good intentions and she relished the warm attention.

I was not brave enough to be in Moosh's room when the sisters said their farewells, but I know that they were unsurprisingly tearful, because Sandra was still glassy-eyed as we drove home and then, later, to the airport.

It had been a truly special, unwished for in our wildest dreams, five days, only slightly spoilt by Sandra sharing, just before going through the airport barrier, "Your Mum is very worried about you. She says that you work too hard and need to look after yourself better. She asked me to tell you that you need to lose weight and she's right: you could do with losing a few pounds."

Thanks!

Sisters.

Clearly they had spoken about the important stuff.

46

The House Sale

Moosh always wanted to keep the house on Shakespeare Road.

She had long accepted that she would never be going back to live there, but she had ideas that Aly or Liam might use it as a base, or even a home, at some nebulous point in the future. More than anything, she kept it because it was her gift from Dad and it had been truly hers.

I had managed to abide by her wishes for almost three years. The refurbishments had been finished in 2007 and I had two different purchasers lined up, one regularly asking me for updates throughout the decoration works and continuing to ask whether Moosh had changed her mind for almost a year. Moosh continued to prevaricate and eventually the interest died off. I was able to hold on to the house, because I paid the bills for Moosh's care out of her savings, her pensions and the allowances that were granted based on her health needs.

The cycle of meetings that had begun when Moosh was

living with us had continued, so that Moosh's needs were regularly reviewed. Moosh always did her best to demonstrate that she would still be able to sprint 100m, if only she could get rid of the pesky wheelchair.

For me, the review meetings were a necessary evil; I needed them to take place. I understood about funding and that, for funding to be received, criteria had to be met and ticked off, allowing calculations to be made. I operated within similar processes at school when trying to secure or retain funding for children with particular needs.

In Moosh's case, I was delighted that the wonderful care that the home provided had lengthened her life far beyond our original three-week expectation, but at each meeting I was in the awful position of hoping that she appeared ill enough to retain her funding. Sometimes she did and sometimes she did not. When she did, I could hold on to her savings against the needs of an uncertain future. When she did not, we would have six months of harvesting a far greater portion of those savings, watching her pot deplete with fretful calculations of how many more months her savings would cover.

In early 2010, one of Moosh's stronger periods coincided with her review meeting.

With clear regret and sympathy for my position the chair informed me that, on this occasion, Moosh's needs did not meet the criteria for funding. I would be able to secure a review if there was a significant change in Moosh's needs, but, for now, she no longer qualified. Looking at Moosh, I had to concede that she was in a good place, not quite up to mounting serious escape bids, but in the meeting, and for weeks before, she had been full of vim and her old engaging sparkle. It was lovely to see, and, in conscience, I would not have given her the funding, either, if it had been my decision.

The only downside to this improved vitality was that I knew that Moosh's savings were evaporating like a receding oasis in a very hot desert.

When I, once again, mooted the possibility that we would need to sell Shakespeare Road to supplement her savings, she surprised me, as she often did, "Alistair, it's time. I'm never going back am I?"

I was expecting an argument or at the very least, a degree of resistance.

The last thing that I was expecting was stoic resignation, so I pressed, largely as salve to my own sense of guilt, "Ma, are you sure? I know you were keeping it for Aly and Liam."

"Needs must, Alistair," she assured me, before adding, "We aren't going to get too much by selling this old body of mine, so you'd better get the best price possible for my house! We need it!"

Entertained by her own humour, she cackled so strenuously that she set off her dyskinetic writhing and slid down in her chair under her table, until her bum was hanging over the floor, her head was where her bum should have been, and her arms were flailing in the air like two flags of surrender.

Her laughter was still pealing, as she wailed, "Don't laugh, you meanie! Help me!"

As I restored her to her seat, I realised with a pang that she looked even tinier than normal, dwarfed in the chair, but there was strength in her words when she repeated, "Yes, it is time."

And so, I embarked on the process of house selling.

In my book, house selling is not given sufficiently weighty recognition in the list of stressful life events. Perhaps some divine force was thinking that, with the risk of Moosh passing away somewhat in abeyance and school pretty much under control after our last inspection, I could do with a stress boost.

Looking back, I am more than a little stunned that I ran pretty much the entire house sale myself, without any unwelcome uxorial disharmony. Her Most Wonderfulness talked with me about which estate agent I would use and about which friends had received good or bad service from the many different house sellers on Bearwood Road, but other than that, knowing that I would see her well intentioned advice as unrequested interference, she kept her oar almost entirely out.

I plumped for using the estate agent through whom we bought our own house. I was stunned that, without even seeing the house, the agent, Matt, declared with admirable certainty that, on Moosh's road, we should set the asking price at £110,000 to give us the wiggle room to achieve the £100,000 that I was hoping for.

Just as noticing the youthfulness of policemen, doctors and teachers is a sign of advancing age, Matt seemed very young to be an estate agent, not to say overly confident, but £100,000 would give an enormous fillip to Moosh's finances, so I was encouraged.

After I had arranged for the garden to be given another tidy up and given the house a thorough spring clean, photos and measurements were taken. House particulars were written up and sent for my approval. I showed them to Moosh, but she wanted nothing to do with the actual sale.

And so, her house was finally on the market.

Nothing. Not a sniff. *No interest, whatsoever!*

I visited both of the families who had wanted to buy Moosh's house back in 2007, telling them that it was now available and the price and inviting them to come for an informal viewing. They did come and were very complimentary about the works that had been carried out, before each admitting that their circumstances had changed and they were no longer looking to buy.

Perturbed and about to fork out another monthly payment for Moosh's care, I visited the estate agent to query the lack of results. Rather sheepishly, Matt admitted that he was not entirely surprised, which, in turn, took me totally by surprise.

"Mark, your mum's house has everything. Three good sized bedrooms. Well refurbished. A lovely garden with lots of space. It should be selling. I think it's the colour."

Despite my worries about the lack of money pouring into Moosh's bank account, I had to laugh, "It is a bit shit, isn't it!"

And I meant quite literally, *shit.*

Moosh was something of a maverick, when she decided to have the outside of her house painted. She was taken by the idea of being a bit different, wanting a colour that would stand out. I like houses that stand out, too, and often look admiringly at the multi-hued Cinque Terre in Italy, promising yearningly that we will visit one day. With Moosh I shared a fondness for the kaleidoscope of colourful houses Her Most Wonderfulness and I had seen in Galway.

The problem was that Moosh chose a tinge of green that defies description without going faecal. The last time that I had seen the shade that Moosh chose to adorn her house was inside Ayesha's nappy, when she was teething. *You almost expected to smell that house!*

When Glen had painted the house, years before, he had opened the tin to stir the paint and asked one last time, "Are you sure you're absolutely sure about this, Mark? Sure sure?"

"Not my house, mate," had been my forlorn reply.

Following Matt's advice to go for 'nice, plain white', and going against Moosh's continued assertions of 'but it is distinctive', I asked Glen to come back to paint the exterior the white that he had always thought it should have been.

Matt was right.

There was interest within three days of the new photograph being displayed in the estate agent window, evidencing the colour change.

In less than a week, Matt had an offer, "It's not quite what you were hoping for Mark: £95,000. But the buyer is in a good position and ready to move in. We could do the deal quickly."

I have never been much of a haggler. When Her Most Wonderfulness reverts to her Indian roots to engage in haggling, enthusiastically channeling her experiences as a teenage market trader on her father's stall in Newcastle-under-Lyme, I tend to scurry off, too embarrassed to watch.

My brain was screaming, "We need £100K! Just walk away!"

And my heart was hoping, "Maybe there'll be other offers."

When I put this to Matt, his view was, "I think this is a

good offer and a good scenario for you, the purchaser is ready to move. There should be other offers, but this one is here, now."

Ultimately, it was Moosh's house and Moosh's money, and so I asked her.

Being a telly addict she momentarily forgot that it was her house that we were talking about and her savings pot at stake and, instead, turned into Noel Edmonds, gravely intoning, "And so the question is: £95,000, deal or no deal?"

She even gave the dramatic pause before clapping: "Deal! Let's not mess the poor girl around. Then we can all stop worrying and get on with our lives."

Despite that boyish appearance, Matt was clearly well versed in his job: the conveyancing took almost no time.

Just before we reached completion, I let Moosh's buyer know that I would like to take my Mum for one last visit to the house to say her goodbyes, and then the house was all hers.

"What is she like?" Moosh wanted to know as we drove the short distance past the cemetery to Shakespeare Road.

"Young, mixed race, single, very friendly," I answered.

"Would I be happy that she is going to be taking over my home?" She asked.

The people that we bought our first house from had been very keen that, out of several couples wanting to buy their home, we were the ones who were successful, as they had taken a shine to us. I think it was something to do with the rapport between me and their giant Doberman and the fact that I was fascinated by their fish tanks. So, I understood that it mattered to Moosh.

"Yes, Ma, I think that she will look after it and turn it

into her type of home, for her and her little boy," I answered, feeling especially connected to this little person, who so often made me chuckle with her ways, but whose sentimentality chimed with my own; we, too, had cared who bought our first 'together home' from us.

As I guided her out of the Zafira's passenger door, in front of the home that she had last lived in almost four years previously, she looked up lovingly (not at me, but at the now dazzlingly white house) and sighed, "I know you didn't like it, but it was mine. All mine."

Despite her uplift in health allowing her to walk to her house, this last time, and climb the two steps, the challenge of the staircase to the first floor was beyond her. She settled for gazing up them for a long moment, before we walked slowly through the long-empty, but now pristine lounge-dining room and into the kitchen where she once again cooed at the tiles that had never been hers to enjoy.

Finally, we stepped out into her garden. Second to being in Church, this had been the physical place that had given her most contentment. We walked as far as she could manage, with her stroking shrubs, naming favourite plants, as if to remind herself, logging them for future reminiscences and urging me to take cuttings or whole clumps of perennials.

And then with a firm nod of her head and a squeeze of my hand she said, "Come on. It's time for her to make this shiny white house her home, for her and her little one. I hope she will love it as much as I have. Let's buy a 'New Home' card for her on our way."

348

47

London To Paris 2010

In January 2010 my interests took me in a new direction, one which took me away from Moosh.

Standing at the funeral of my friend, Chris, reading my eulogy to him, I suddenly decided that I wanted to do the London To Paris bike ride to raise money in his memory.

There was a logic to this. Knowing that he had cancer, Chris had hoped to take part in the charity ride the year before, but was forced to withdraw as his illness took greater hold. Brilliantly, his son and other male relatives climbed into their saddles to take his place. Reading his eulogy, I felt moved to take up the baton from them to raise money for the hospice that had provided wonderful care for him.

There were, however, small but not inconsiderable obstacles to be overcome, if I was to see this wish through: I had never ridden further than ten miles in my life; I did not have a functioning bike; I was very unfit; and most importantly, I spent the greater portion of my free time with Moosh.

In honesty, bikes had never truly held any fascination for

me. As a teenager, like all of my friends, I had a bike, but most of the time bikes were not for going for rides of any significant distance; they were just for getting about. I do have a nostalgic, vivid memory from my boarding school years of a bike ride along a ridge in Staffordshire looking down on a cloud filled valley. But, I have others of dismally trailing far behind a friend who had loaned me a manky bike, cursing that there was no fun in it. I sold my last 'teenager bike' at the age of seventeen, to raise funds to go on a school trip to France and Italy and, although I did buy bikes at different times as an adult, in a bid to commit to exercise, the flesh was weak and my bum never quite took to the discomfort. The urge to take part in this charity bike ride ignited an enthusiasm where none had previously existed.

When I decided that I would like to do London To Paris, I did actually possess a bike, bought at Chris's encouragement, which I had ridden to school precisely three times in five years. However, it was now a neglected, rust addled hulk in the shed, unlikely to carry me the three miles to Handsworth, let alone the three hundred to Paris. I guiltily cleaned cobwebs and grime from the bike and rubbed away as much rust as possible, before taking it to a bike repair shop to be serviced, but the mechanic, who checked it over for me, shook her head accusingly, pointing to a broken tooth on one of the cogs and advised me to buy a replacement bike. That was easily remedied on a trip to Hawks. I explained what I was planning and was shown a shiny, silver Mongoose Crossway tourer, which I loved (for its comfy saddle) and bought.

I have often flirted with the idea of fitness, but never been able to find it in me to sustain the level of commitment required to maintain it. For the last decade it had been easy to hide behind the workload of being a head teacher and complain that I could not find the time to exercise. Knowing that I should commit, I made sporadic forays into gym membership and, when I go, I love it (although the thing I love most is the saunas). Inevitably I falter, but I retain my gym membership as a prod to my conscience: I have paid my current, rarely used membership for so long that I believe each actual visit to the gym costs me roughly £400.

The training plan sent by the bike ride organisers was strenuous. I had signed up a little late and was a tad behind the other fund raisers, who had already begun their preparations.

What lay ahead was four months of increasingly demanding slog.

When I hesitantly told Moosh about my urge to ride to Paris, I was expecting reluctant agreement on the condition that I came to see her at the same time each week.

Once again, I had underestimated her, as nothing could have been further from the truth.

"You must do this ride!" she exclaimed.

"Really? It will mean quite a lot of time away from here," I cautioned, gesticulating around her small room and at her.

"Don't you worry. I remember how much you loved working with Chris. He was your hero," she stated emphatically. Then, with her hand placed gently on mine, continued, "You'll enjoy doing this in his memory, and it will give us lots to talk about when you visit."

"That's true. I can tell you about aches and pains and you can tell me about ancient remedies for them: I can already hear you suggesting poultices of eye of toad and tail of newt to be rubbed vigorously on my aching buttocks!" I joked.

"If you're going to tease me, I won't ask you to write the cheque for £100 that I was about to sponsor you," she grinned.

"Blimey, Ma, that's a lot of your money!" I protested, half-heartedly, knowing that a three-digit donation would be a great beginning for my sponsorship page.

"I know, but I want to. It is a great cause," she insisted. "Besides, you never listened to your Auntie Sandra, when she passed on my message about needing to lose weight. I think this might finally motivate you to get yourself fit."

Caught between my joy at my burgeoning fund-raising pot and my wounded pride, I opted for a vaguely hurt expression, which only served to magnify Moosh's smug, winning smirk.

"Fair," I conceded.

Alongside Her Most Wonderfulness, Moosh became one of my staunchest supporters.

Over the months that followed, she became utterly absorbed as I ticked off each week's targets and generously applauded each new gain, and became quite a brutal armchair personal trainer. When I initially quailed at the jump from my previous PB distance of ten miles for a single ride to the thirty demanded by the programme, it was Moosh who reverted to her default setting that I can do anything I set my mind to.

In my experience, all loving mothers hold this belief about their children, but I contend that the level of unrealism that Moosh was prone to displaying far outstrips that of any other mother. This was perhaps best exemplified during the

Moscow Summer Olympics in 1980 when, as a seventeen-year-old, I developed the most ardent crush for the Soviet Union gymnast, Yelena Davydova. Far from counselling me that Yelena was thousands of miles away, spoke Russian and probably spent her entire life slaving away in the gym, Moosh encouraged me to take up gymnastics, become an Olympian and go get to know her. When I laughingly pointed out that I had precisely zero gymnastic experience and was not keen on heights or spinning, Moosh derided my defeatist attitude, repeating her maternal mantra that I could achieve anything I was willing to strive for, but nothing that I did not have the nerve to attempt.

I took to mapping my routes on my laptop, so that I could show her where I had been, with an accompaniment of photographs taken on the ride and souvenirs that I bought for her, usually postcards. It was almost as if my trips took her out of her nursing home room and out into the countryside and to neighbouring villages, towns and cities. She loved to hear about Hagley, Belbroughton, Stourport, Bridgenorth, Worcester, Evesham and Warwick, everywhere my two wheels took me.

Despite her voluble support, she was not above laughing at some of my tribulations. She was highly entertained when I rode over brambles out on the canal path on the way back from Tamworth, fifteen miles from home, only to find that I had a puncture repair kit but no pump and had to walk several miles before pleading at a lawn mower repair shop for the loan of a pump. She was just as tickled when I suffered a blow out on the Uttoxeter ring road, midway through an arduous ride through the Peak District, and hitched a fortuitous ride home in an RAC van. But she howled at her belly-laughing best the day I was splattered from helmet to pedal by a malodorous muck spreader - I did briefly question my maternal lineage.

That said, she turned into a lioness the day that a lager bottle, near full, was launched at me from a car window on a back road between Stratford-upon-Avon and Leamington Spa. Admittedly she was an ageing, toothless lioness with unreliable dentures, but, if she could have caught up with the young men in that car, they would have resembled *Zebra Tartare*.

She enjoyed being updated about how much sponsorship had been pledged and how much received. She urged everyone that she came into contact with to sponsor me. I had to forbid her from pressurising the staff at the home to contribute, as they were her unfairly captive audience. When Alex organised a fund-raising gig, she donated again, despite her disappointment that her immobility prevented her from joining us on the night.

In addition to mentally taking her on virtual tours away from the home, my training had two other benefits that Moosh greatly approved of.

Firstly, as well as my ever-increasing weekend training rides, I began to cycle to and from school. Several evenings a week, I ensured that my route home, however long I made it, took me past her window. The staff were always happy for me to wheel my bike in, however mud splattered, and lean it against the wall outside her room to pop in for a chat. However short that visit was, however rained on or sweaty I was, it brought a smile to Moosh's face and a fresh dose of encouragement for me.

Secondly, my weight loss delighted Moosh. She was

genuinely (and correctly) concerned that my sedentary lifestyle – office bound at work and often too exhausted for much in the way of movement at the end of each day – was harming me. Being on a bike melted thirty-five pounds of excess weight from my frame, meaning for me that I did not have to carry it round with me on my bike, and for Moosh that I was giving myself a chance of better health.

I had huge support for the bike ride at school and from friends and family, but Moosh was my greatest encourager and follower. Hearing about each weekend's rides added a new dimension to our conversations.

When the time came for the bike ride itself, I was under a strict directive to take photographs of everything and to come back and tell her all about the adventures.

Luckily, several of the friends I made on the trip were under similar instructions, so we stopped often, alongside fields of poppies, serene mill ponds and chocolate box chateaux, but the two pictures that Moosh loved the most were one of me holding my bike above my head in front of the Eiffel Tower and one of a group of us standing outside Sacre Coeur, where I had lit a candle for her and one for Chris.

She was deeply touched when I told her that on Day 2 of the ride, I cycled much of the morning solo, with only she and Chris chatting inside my head (although the jab of her elbow was hard, when I chuckled that, in my imaginary conversations, Chris had spoken far more sense than she).

Even approaching the age of forty-seven, there was something enormously rewarding about witnessing Moosh's pride in me. London To Paris is not the longest bike ride in the world, but I raised £6000 for the hospice that had looked after Chris.

Moosh was deeply proud of that, and I basked in her approbation.

48

Pneumonia

The summer holiday after my London To Paris challenge was one of those selfishly blissful ones for Ranjit and me.

Comparatively speaking, Moosh was hale and hearty. There would be no hundred-mile bike rides or ultra-wheel chair-challenges for her, but she was enjoying a period when her body was doing more of the limited range of things that she asked it to. Meaning that she could make it to the loo unaided, potter around her room without harming herself and tend to her plants without them crashing to the floor. For perspective, however, the 7 metres to the nurse's station would have been several steps too far, even with her Zimmer.

Her greatest delight of July was the return of her ability to write. Prior to the onset of Parkinson's, Moosh had always had perfect, precise handwriting in a beautiful, almost delicate, cursive script. She was an enthusiastic writer, penning lengthy letters to friends. Having never been the most consistently outward person, letter writing afforded Moosh a way of communicating with her small group of friends that the telephone never did. Moosh would much sooner pick up a pen to drop into the life of a friend, than pick up the handset. There was a freedom in talking through writing that simply was not there through the phone. By limiting her muscular control of her hand, and therefore a pen, Parkinson's had robbed her of that communication.

Moosh was determined to write. Her collection of pens had remained on her table, unused, but an optimistic possibility. Arriving at her door on the last Saturday in June, I found her hunched over her small table, head bowed, deep in concentration. She did not look up, so intensely focussed was she on the sheet of paper before her, pinned in place by her left arm.

Sidling around in front of her, I could see her head tilted, her tongue gripped between clamped dentures and, to my pleased surprise, her hand holding a black fibre tip pen. The sheet of paper was covered with words, in various states of legibility. None came close to her flowing penmanship, some were wiggly lines, others were disjointed and childlike. It was a long way from being a letter to a friend, but, in a few of the attempts, the eight letters of my name could clearly be discerned, repeated.

Registering my presence, Moosh covered the sheet.

Guessing her intent, I allowed her secrecy and got on with unpacking goodies and setting up Scrabble, before saying, "I'm dead impressed. I knew you could control your pen enough to do word searches, but writing words is a huge step."

"I haven't tried for a while, because I was frustrated, but I like trying to make my body do things that Parkinson's doesn't want me to. I'll keep practising," she beamed. "Now, stop wasting time. Let's play."

A little over a week later, when I collected her for another birthday Chinese take away, Moosh proudly presented me with an envelope with my name emblazoned in a legible print. The message inside was spidery to such an extreme that arachnophobes would have fled, but it was all her own work and I could read every word.

Bless! Her face was the personification of triumph: she was back to writing.

For me, I was on a triple whammy.

Moosh was in a good place. I still basked in the cycle challenge afterglow, both the money raised and the fact that I was physically healthier than I had been for years. At school, there was definitely no possibility of an impending inspection – I would not miscalculate that ever again. This left my mind freer to relax and my body much more willing to enjoy life.

For Ranjit, all of these things made me much more pleasant to be around. To cap it all, she was excited about Alex's decision that he was finally going to university after *three* gap years. We were set for a good summer, with the delightful prospect of a fortnight in our favourite patch of Languedocian wine country. We had made all the usual preparations of Aly being on call to come down, if Moosh needed her.

As it turned out, Moosh did need her.

While I was happily swanning off on a hired bike to pootle 40 miles round the Etang de Thau, Moosh was hit by a nasty chest infection which rapidly became an even more concerning bout of pneumonia. Dangerous enough for her to be hospitalised.

As arranged, I initially knew nothing of this and we continued to bask in Mediterranean sunshine, while Aly fielded the call from the nursing home to alert her, first to the concerns of chestiness and the resultant GP visits, and then to the need for hospitalisation. Only at the point of Moosh being kept in at Sandwell General, did Aly intrude apologetically on our holiday.

"Al, I didn't want to worry you unnecessarily, but now that they are keeping Moosh in, I thought that I had best put you in the picture," she explained, before admitting, "To be honest, she looks like shit at the moment.

"But you must not come home. Moosh would hate it if you cut your holiday short. We are visiting and Arun and Alex are going to visit too, now that I have let them know. They were really worried, but they have been great. You can be very proud of them.

"Just promise me that you will stay where you are."

With Aly's reassurances, Ranjit and I agreed not to change our travel plans, and enjoyed, more mutedly, our second week in the sun, checking back with Aly and with Alex and Arun.

Phoning Arun, I could hear his unstated discomfort at visiting a hospital, his unexpressed sense of uselessness in the face of Moosh's weakness, but I was encouraged by the maturity that he showed in his assertive assurance of, "We've got this, Dad. We'll visit and the hospital are saying that she is improving. We'll see you next week. I just wish Grandma would be nicer to Aly."

He would say no more.

Neither would Aly, who remained tight lipped, when I attempted to quiz her.

Upon returning home, we made for the hospital and Moosh.

And for a third time, our lives reverted to the grind of feeding the ever-greedy hospital parking metre, keeping ward visiting hours, forming relationships with a new set of medical staff and keeping tabs on developments.

I was not familiar with Sandwell General Hospital and so was, initially, a little out of sorts as we orientated ourselves, but we quickly found a routine, which revolved around two priorities: being there and bringing food. Moosh decided that the food was execrable and so we took to ferrying in doggy bags from our meals at home and putting together bespoke packages at her request.

It completely slipped my mind to explore Arun's reference to something having happened between Moosh and Aly.

It was very clear that Moosh was on an upward curve by the time we arrived back in the UK. The talk of a 'pleasing recovery' and 'careful monitoring to be certain that your mother is out of the woods' indicated that she had been in a much more precarious position than the smiling, little, Yoda type creature that we were faced with each time we visited, often twice a day.

I was a firm respecter of pneumonia, having unexpectedly found myself coming round in ICU, almost exactly five years previously. As I had regained consciousness, I was aware of Teresa consoling Ranjit as she grappled with the possibility that I might die. As a result, I recognised that Moosh had been in very grave danger and was delighted to find that she was well on the road to recovery, from the pneumonia at least.

It was also clear that Alex and Arun were delighted to have us re-assume the bulk of the hospital run burden. They had done their bit to man the barricades in our absence, but Alex needed to get back to preparing for his imminent departure to Oxford to study music, and Arun just hated hospitals, so would not go again. We had had our vacation and were as happy as it is possible to be when faced with resuming the filial responsibility of hospital visits.

Alyson left us to it.

I did not challenge her. She had done her part, being there, when I was not.

It only slipped out, a couple of months later, how terrified Aly had been about the graveness of Moosh's situation and how abominably Moosh had treated her.

Moosh's condition had been sufficiently dire for her to be allocated a private room on the ground floor. While Ranjit swanned around markets in different Herault villages and I snorkelled in limpid seas, both of us beneath a blazing sun in a cerulean sky, Aly had uncomplainingly travelled down repeatedly; she could navigate her way from the car park to the door of Moosh's room with her eyes closed.

On the day of her last visit, Aly had driven down with Jess and they had duly arrived at the room, to find the door open and the room vacated. There was not even a bed. Aly was apoplectic, being familiar with the repeated scenario of morbidly ill patients shuffling off their mortal coil in Sheldon Block, in the months that Moosh had been there. On one of her visits to the geriatric ward, Aly had arrived the day after the woman in the bed opposite had died in the night . .

362

. her bed had been removed. Seeing Moosh's room empty now panicked Aly and she raced off in search of a nurse and information.

Her relief at learning that Moosh had merely been taken for an MRI scan and was still of this world, was immense. She and Jess busied themselves with sorting through Moosh's cupboard, which they now realised did in fact contain her clothes and washbag. Finding themselves not having to grieve, they instead let Alex and Arun know that they were at the hospital, found tea, coffee and sustenance at the café and waited, gratefully.

Moosh was duly returned to the room, with Aly bursting to greet the mother who, only shortly before, she had thought lost forever. Jess was also bouncing at the reprieve.

From Moosh there was precisely nothing. Not one word. Not a look. No reciprocation. No acknowledgement of Aly and Jess's presence. She was conscious. She responded to the nurses. But to Aly she was frostily unresponsive, even when Aly tried to kiss her in greeting. The nurses, embarrassed, made themselves scarce. Moosh completely and coldly ignored Aly and Jess in stony silence for forty-five minutes. Stung and confused, having driven 200 hundred miles to be rebuffed and looked through, Aly was at a loss.

When Alex and Arun arrived, as they had planned with Aly, Moosh instantly transformed into their besotted grandmother, grateful for their presence and keen to hear how they were. She enthusiastically enquired about Alex's progress in his preparations for university. She became, in Aly's devastated words, 'the life and soul of the party'. Admittedly it was a party in a hospital room where she was extremely weak, but she radiated her adoration of two of her grandsons, while continuing to pointedly shun Aly and Jess.

Aly and Jess drove back to Loftus.

Even years later, when I asked her about her visits to Moosh, the pain of that day was nakedly visible on Aly's face. The injustice of it still rankled.

However, in the days and weeks after it happened, Aly did what she had always done when Moosh was hospitalised. She communicated with the hospital to check on Moosh's progress and, as the risk from the pneumonia first reduced and then retreated, her focus reverted to securing updates about Moosh's Parkinson's related difficulties.

She did not visit for months, but she emailed me and phoned to keep me abreast of her findings and concerns. The pneumonia was no longer an issue, and Moosh was back at the nursing home, but the speech and language therapist had identified that Moosh's swallow was very weak, leaving her at risk of choking on the limited food that she was eating. Alongside the weak swallow was a very feeble cough, which lacked any umph. I had not realised that coughing was important, but Aly enlightened me by explaining that humans need to be able to cough to clear our airways. With Moosh's seemingly pathetic cough ability, she would be unable to help herself out of trouble 'if anything went down the wrong way'. In such an event, Moosh's frailty would limit her capacity to help herself or to attract help. Based on information from the speech and language therapist, Aly agonised over the relative benefits of a pureed or mashed diet, and made herself learn more about strength of swallow and cough than I ever wanted to know.

Although I was entirely uninterested in adding to the

research being done by Aly, I was terrified at the thought of losing Moosh, but, yet again, I was preparing myself to do so. I repeatedly found myself pondering how many brushes with death an octogenarian could cope with - I was not sure how many I could.

My journeys home from school, a daily interval of alone time in which my brain would subconsciously flit far and wide as I drove, were regularly intruded upon by tortured thoughts about whether Moosh would prefer for her struggles to be over.

Often, at these unbidden broodings, I would turn my wheel and nip to the nursing home, just to be near her for a few minutes.

49

I'm Kay

Despite ostensibly being perfectly comfortable in her own company, back in her little room at the nursing home, and still persisting, as ever, in her refusal to interact with the other residents, Moosh contented and sometimes consoled herself with the certain knowledge that I would visit.

There were, however, other visitors who filled Moosh with joy, unexpected ones from her past.

Sandra had been one.

One day, I answered the phone to an unfamiliar woman's voice, asking if she was speaking to Alistair and introducing herself as Kay. Trawling as rapidly as possible through my memories, the only Kay that I could conjure was a workmate from my first school, and, even to me unskilled ear, the voice on the phone was older, plus my friend knew me as Mark.

The woman continued, "I'm a friend of your mother: Kay Wood from Guernsey. I was married to John, Patsy's father."

The penny didn't merely drop: it plummeted, crashing into my befuddled cranium, where my brain was struggling weakly to comprehend exactly how Kay Wood could be speaking to me on the phone. Guernsey was the key clue: Kay was Moosh's 'step-stepmother'. Her husband, John, had been married to Moosh's mother, Nora, becoming Moosh's stepfather, despite her absence on the other side of the world. Moosh referred to him, fondly, as Pops. In sorting through paper's from Moosh's treasured antique desk at Shakespeare Road, I had found the kindest letters from Pops written to Moosh in Malaya, sent at a time in her life when he could not possibly have even met her yet, because Moosh only returned to England in 1964. After Nora passed away in the sixties, John had married Kay, making her Moosh's step-stepmother.

Moosh's early life is a long, convoluted and painful story that I am still unearthing, but which I hope to write one day. I must confess that I had assumed Kay to be dead: I knew that Moosh had an address for her, but she had never mentioned any contact or communication between the two of them.

Trying to cover my astonishment at holding a conversation with a not-ghost, I wittered, "Kay, of course! Thank you for explaining. I'm so sorry for not placing you! Mum is not going to believe this! How are you and how can I help?"

Relief washed down the phone line, "Geraldine's OK, then? I was worried that she might not be. Is she still at the nursing home on Bearwood Road?"

Poleaxed, this time: "Yes. Yes, she is still there. You've been in contact with her? When? Gosh, I'm sorry, I had no idea. It's one surprise after another and I'm in a bit of a dither."

"Yes, Christmas cards. Birthday cards. Phone calls, before she became too ill," Kay explained with such warmth that I fell just a little bit in love, though, given the tenuous family connection, I was sure that was unfitting. "Nothing recently, though. How is she?"

"She's very up and down, Kay. More down than up, recently, to be absolutely honest. She's been very weak, since having pneumonia in the summer and we feared the worst. She's rallied a little – stubborn or determined, I can't decide which. She will be delighted to hear that you were asking after her. Little things like that really lift her spirits," I answered, as my brain finally came up to speed.

There was a short pause, before Kay continued, "Can I ask, do I call you Alistair or Mark? It's just that Geraldine refers to you as Alistair, but she gave me your name as Mark with your number, when she was coming to live with you. I'm a little confused."

"In the world of confused, I think I'm streets ahead of you, this evening, but almost everyone calls me Mark, nowadays," I laughed. "It's all my Dad's fault and a very long story."

She laughed along with me, "Maybe you could tell me the story, when we meet."

"I'm sorry? Meet?" Kay laughed even more heartily, with quite an earthy undertone. I really was becoming rather smitten by a lady, who had to be, I calculated, at the very least of my mother's vintage. "Are you coming to Birmingham?"

Just to revert to complete dullard mode, I added, "From Guernsey?" as if the Channel Islands orbit the Earth somewhere out past Uranus.

"I'm here already!" Kay declared between what was becoming entirely inappropriately endearing gales of mirth, leaving me in no doubt that she could imagine the affect her announcement was having. "In Quinton with my friend, Bridie. Sorry to add to the surprises for the night! I

368

was wondering whether you could arrange for me to visit Geraldine, while I am here."

"You're staying with Bridie? Or do you need somewhere to stay?"

Innate politeness momentarily trumped the reeling in my mind. Moosh had so few living relatives and here was one, who I thought had gone entirely, offering to visit!

I was getting carried away, anticipating Moosh's reinvigoration as I visualised taking Kay to her, but I managed to offer, "We have lots of space and a room ready."

"No, no, but thank you. Bridie has a bed for me here, so I will be staying with her for a couple of nights," Kay assured me.

It being midweek, I was inwardly grateful to not be doing a rapid tidy of the office cum guest bedroom, which was once again in need of a thorough going over, but Kay brought me back to her, "I'm sorry that I haven't given you more warning, but do you think I could visit, tomorrow, and could Bridie come too? She would like to."

"Tomorrow?"

Rapidly, I visualised my diary pages for the next couple of days, but knew that whatever had been there would quickly become secondary to placing Kay in Moosh's room.

"That would be fabulous. I can pick the two of you up. What time works for you?"

"I don't want to put you to any trouble," Kay insisted. "We can get a cab."

"Kay," I stopped her. "Of all the things I could possibly be doing with my life tomorrow, believe me, none will be better than taking you to see Mum. I usually get home from work at 6:00pm, but can leave earlier. What time shall I collect

369

you?"

"That is so kind of you." Again, her voice exuded warmth, "How about 6:30pm? We will have eaten, but we are old girls now and will need to be home at a sensible time."

When Kay gave me Bridie's address, I was, again, staggered, as she was so close that I could have walked there in the time that it had taken us to hold the conversation.

Knowing that I would have happily walked round immediately to find out more about Kay's tenuous links with Moosh, I reluctantly ended the call with, "I'll be there at 6:30pm. Mum is going to be so happy to see you. Thank you so much for calling. Night night."

Having, most uncharacteristically, managed not to plague the phone conversation with a barrage of interrupting questions, Ranjit laughed happily to see me absolutely abuzz, "She sounded lovely. This will do Geraldine the world of good."

The powerful hug she gave me added a silent, "I'm so pleased for you. Both of you."

50

The Pen Factory

Beyond excited, and having no idea what to expect, I set off to collect Moosh's step-stepmother.

The road off which Bridie's sheltered accommodation sat was one of my favourite rat-runs behind the busy arterial junction of the Wolverhampton and Hagley roads, but it took me a while to find the exact address, leaving me slightly breathless as I arrived to act as chauffeur. However, my sense of arriving only just on time quickly evaporated as the door of one of the maisonettes opened to reveal two ladies of an older generation, clearly ready to go visiting. They were smartly dressed and positively twinkling. Despite their evident age (which my particular brand of masculine vagueness about female ages placed somewhere in the 60 to 90 age-bracket), they exuded the girlish giggliness of a friendship that, I would quickly learn, stretched back to their school days.

I slowed the rush of my arrival to a pace suitable to helping dual walking stick wielding Bridie to climb into my Zafira.

Kay required no assistance, almost leaping into the rear of the car to sit next to her pal.

She covered her unobtrusive checking that Bridie was buckled up and comfortable, by asking, "So why are you Mark not Alistair?"

So I began to tell her the story of Dad setting off to the registry office with Alistair Mark in his head, but, having had a drink on the way, being inspired to plump for Mark Alistair, without Moosh's permission. The resultant fallout left me called by my middle name, her choice, but I had chosen to use Mark in preference to my teenage friends' nickname for me inspired by the 70s cartoon 'Crystal Tipps And Alistair'.

Only too late did I realise that I had to utter the punchline of "No teenage boy wants their nickname to be 'Crystal Tits'!" to my very ladylike car guests.

The unexpectedly raucous hoots from the backseat broke the ice, and seeing that Kay was satisfied with the seatbelt situation, I hid my blushes by asking, "Are we ready to go?"

"Oh yes," chirped Bridie, still chuckling. "It is lovely to be taken out!"

As we drove along the Hagley Road and onto Bearwood Road, we fell into that rapid exchange of 'getting to know you' details: the trip from Guernsey had been pleasant; Ranjit and I had been married since '87 and had three children; Kay and Bridie had been friends at Holly Lodge Grammar School; Kay regretted that she didn't get over to visit Bridie as often as she would like and it was now too difficult for Bridie to travel far; they applauded the fact that I was a head teacher and joked that they had better behave.

All the while, their eyes were switching between mine in the rear-view mirror and the passing urbanscape.

"It's so much busier than the last time I was here and so many charity shops," remarked Kay, "but the bears are still there."

Craning her neck, she pointed upwards, as we approached the traffic lights, to the 3D decorations below the domed roof of the Bear Tavern.

"I bet most people passing by never look up to see those wonderful bears," offered Bridie, a tad wistfully.

Searching further ahead, Kay asked, "Is Bearwood School still here? I went there as a girl."

"It is!" I exclaimed. "You lived this close to where I live now? Several of our friends have taught there. Lots of our friends' children went there too, although ours went to Abbey."

"Up on the hill in the woods?" Kay asked and continued, "Yes, I had friends who went there too, but Bearwood was closer to us."

"Near here?" I asked, as we passed the imposing, red brick structure of Kay's old school with her peering out nostalgically, appearing to be awash with a flood of memories.

"Yes, just down towards the old pen factory."

Before she could elaborate, Bridie was excitedly tugging her sleeve and pointing at a building that I knew as the snooker club, where Arun had enjoyed several years of football presentation nights.

"Look, the ice rink!"

"Bearwood had an ice rink? Its own ice rink? You're kidding me!" I slowed briefly to stare, utterly astonished. An ice rink in Bearwood!

"Oh yes, it was very popular! We had such good times there, speeding round, showing the young ones how to do it. Remember Kay? The looks on their faces!"

It was Bridie's turn to glow and drift off on a wave of memory, "It's been so many things, that building: a cinema, when we were teenagers; a theatre; the ice rink; always popular, always a place that lots of us would go to with our friends."

It was wonderful to look afresh at a building that I had always thought was sadly dilapidated and in real danger of crumbling. The gilded prism of reminiscences were bringing such a smile to Bridie's face, causing the years to flee. An ice rink in Bearwood - who would have thought?

As we approached the fork with Waterloo Road, I asked Kay, "Are we close to where you lived? We haven't passed it?"

"No, we aren't quite there yet," she smiled in response, pointing ahead. "I was born in Wellington Road, just down there on the left."

"Never!" I exclaimed, not for the first time.

As we passed the opening of Wellington, coming to a stop at the lights, I nodded ahead, "You were born just two roads from where Mum is now living! Isn't that a strange quirk of fate?"

"That is the site of the old pen factory! You remember, don't you, Bridie?" Kay exclaimed.

As we drove the last few hundred metres to the nursing home and parked up, Bridie gave me a potted history of British Pens Limited, harking back to an era when Smethwick was a thriving industrial hub.

With gusto, she explained, "Birmingham and the Black

Country manufactured all manner of goods, pens being one speciality. There was a time when hundreds, maybe even a thousand, people worked here making nibs. Fiddly things to make, by all accounts."

"And now it's a nursing home," prompted Kay, kindly, as I climbed out to open the doors for them.

I buzzed in and we made our way to the desk, where I explained that Kay and Bridie had come to visit Moosh, bringing a rush of enthusiasm from one of my favourite Sikh carers, whose name, unforgivably, I never learned.

"Oh Bhaji, how exciting! She will be so pleased. Would you like some tea?"

At my grateful nod, the beaming carer whispered, "Go on in, surprise Geraldine. I will bring some tea, when she gets over the shock."

She followed to capture the best view from just outside the door, as I shielded Kay from Moosh's sight. Moosh had heard us approaching, but had been focussed on the telly, so her eyes were owlish as she looked up at me, both smiling and instantly enquiring. She still looked grey and weak, but was pleased to see me.

"Hello, Ma, I've brought someone to see you, well, some people actually," I greeted her, stepping aside and further into the room.

Moosh's recognition was instant, "Kay!"

Then tears, as she raised her arms and attempted to rise, Kay preventing the need by leaning in to embrace her.

Bridie rested her weight on her sticks, smiling broadly with shimmering eyes. The nameless carer leant on the door post, suffused with an enchanted grin, her hands clasped in a one clap round of unobtrusive applause. I clenched my jaw against the very real possibility of becoming a blubbering washout and basked in the joy of the moment, etching the image into my mind's eye to be treasured.

I had intended to stay with them to share in their reacquaintance and to share in their memories, but as Kay released her embrace to introduce Bridie to Moosh, I felt slightly overwhelmed and confined in the small room. I decided to give these three ladies space and time to share some tea and some nattering. I explained this to them and, although they encouraged me to stay, I made to take my leave.

Kay followed me and urged, "Don't feel that you should stay away for too long, but thank you for thinking of giving us a little while together."

She then continued, "Could I ask a very cheeky favour? What with Bridie and I catching up all day, I didn't manage to buy some chocolates for Geraldine. Is there anywhere close by that you could buy a nice box? Does she still like dark chocolate?"

Just that snippet of Moosh's preference for the bitter thrill of dark chocolate, spoke of a shared relationship, however fleeting, that I had never known about, and of a shared regard. I took the proffered £10 note, delighted that Moosh would have this time with this lady, who was so evidently fond of her. As I headed out into the evening, I had a pronounced spring in my step, very different from the sadness that had typified my gait on recent visits.

When I returned, armed with the largest box of Black Magic that I had been able to find, gales of laughter led me down the corridor to Moosh's room.

She was unrecognisable, as if someone had re-inflated her and filled her, brim-full, with joy and the spark of life. The three of them welcomed me into the room and the box of chocolates was opened, as fresh tea arrived courtesy of the same carer, who was still grinning.

Above the carer's smile, her eyes shone with delighted tears as she murmured, "This is so good for her, Bhaji, can they come every week?"

I have long regretted that I went in search of chocolates, instead of staying to witness the reconnection between Moosh and Kay.

By the time I returned they were well into talking about the present, so I did not hear about Pops, or how they had kept contact without me knowing, or how often the two of them had met one another in their lives. Kay was not on Moosh's 'When I Die, You Must Call These People' list. Given that this was the first time that I had met Kay, I calculated that the number of their meetings must have been few, but there was something about their interaction that was perceptibly rare in its specialness. Maybe it was as simple as mutual regard, or perhaps it was that Kay, too young to be Moosh's mother, had chosen to genuinely care about her 'step-step daughter'. Whatever I was in the presence of, its effect on Moosh was inestimably uplifting. I wanted to bottle it against the hard times that I knew were imminent.

I think the lovely carer felt the specialness too: she was rapt.

Despite her desperate desire to remain awake to lengthen Kay's visit, and the willingness of the carers to allow us to stay, excitement gave way to fatigue and, eventually, Kay,

Bridie and I took our leave with a round of emotional hugs and wishes.

Once again, I was party to a farewell, which all participants knew would, in all likelihood, be the last.

It was utterly crap and boundlessly beautiful all at once.

As I started the ignition in the car park, I offered my fulsome thanks to both Bridie and Kay.

And then in an ingenious scheme to extend our time together and slough off the mutual melancholy, I suggested, "How about we go and look at your birthplace, Kay?"

"Could we? That would be lovely!" came the unfettered reply in stereo.

As we sat in the elbow of Wellington Road staring up at her childhood home, Kay said, "We had good years here and I have such fond memories of our times, including all those times with you, Bridie.

"It's so lovely to come back and to see Geraldine. She had such a difficult early life. I never truly understood what happened, but it must have been devastating to be away from a mother who was still alive.

"Geraldine has always been a loving soul, but there was a gulf in her life until her grandchildren came. She loves them so. It makes me realise how lucky we were, Bridie, having our fun here, with our families around us."

Bridie murmured her agreement, "We were lucky."

And then continued, "It was so lovely to meet your Mum, Mark. Thank you. She is very grateful for everything you do for her, you know. She worries about you trying to balance everything: her, home, school and she worries that you work too hard."

Embarrassed by the praise, but gratified also, I deflected "Did she also say that she worries that I'm getting fat?"

To renewed howls of laughter and strenuous denials, I asked, "Where next? Home? Or revisiting memory lane?"

"Could you take us to see Geraldine's house?" Kay suggested, tentatively. "I always wanted to visit her there."

"Of course," I replied: this experience just kept me smiling.

And so I set off for Shakespeare Road, almost instantly accompanied by Bridie and Kay's recollections, "Oh, The Old Chapel! We were very daring, as young women, going there for our first drink. Isn't it one of the very oldest buildings in the area? Hundreds of years old."

As we passed Uplands Cemetery, Kay said, "Geraldine told us that your father, David, is buried here."

I always experience inexplicable, ghostly tingles on my spine, when I drive that short stretch of road. Kay's comment turned the tingles to jangles, as I marvelled at how much the three of them had shared in my absence.

"Yes, Mum wanted Dad brought here to be buried, as they were a long way down the route of purchasing the house here. Dad had lived in so many places since his boyhood, but none of them had ever become a home with roots, so she brought him to where she could visit him, easily. Ranjit and I always wished that we had simply taken on Mum's mortgage in Shrewsbury, as she left her friends and her church community behind."

"But she is happy that she is close to you, *here*." Kay offered gentle but emphatic reassurance.

As we continued towards Shakespeare Road, Bridie asked, "Mark, we are very close to our old school. Would you mind taking us to see what it looks like?"

I think that I would have agreed to drive around the entire No 11 bus route, if it meant spending more time in the company of those two wonderful women, and so it was that, after a brief stop outside the house that Dad bought for Moosh, but never lived in himself, and Kay confirming from their conversation that Moosh had enjoyed her time there, we drove another half a mile and parked outside Holly Lodge Grammar School for Girls, as it had been back in their day.

I told them that I knew it more recently as the venue for Rock School, a project for aspiring musicians from several local secondary schools, where Alex cut his juvenile guitarist teeth. I lost them for a little while, as they reverted to their teenage selves, waxing lyrical about friends and clothes and dancing and the boys before Pops. It was a very simple pleasure to hear their spiritedly bubbling recollections.

As I reluctantly drove them home, far later than I had planned with school looming in the morning, I passed down the other side of the cemetery, and fascinated by their shared historical knowledge asked, "Was GKN as big as I've heard? The recreation ground is down through there. Arun plays football here and we've had some wonderful evenings in the Rec."

With that, Bridie was off and running with an almost encyclopaedic recount of all things Guest, Keen & Nettleford Ltd, employer of thousands of Smethwick workers in the 20th Century. Supplemented by some diversionary discourse extolling the virtues of the Mitchells & Butlers brewers, Bridie's history of Smethwick kept us going all the way back to me parking the Zafira outside her home. She was a veritable mine of historical knowledge – I should have gone back to capture and record some more of her stories.

Our farewells were fond, sincere and heartfelt.

I spent just that one evening with Kay and Bridie, but I have basked in the memory of that night so many times in the intervening years. It was, without a doubt, one of the best of my life; there was the gold dust of enchantment in it. Kay was one of those rare, special people, and Bridie was a most fabulous sidekick, and I had fallen in love with both of them.

Even as I write and re-read this, I feel enormous gratitude for those hours of unanticipated elation and wonderfully welcome warmth that they brought to Moosh.

51

The Car Park

My darkness came with no warning.

On almost any day of my life, on any car journey, if I am parking, I will reverse into a space, always wanting to be able to drive forwards when I am leaving. But, on the last day of the October half-term holiday my Zafira stood stationary, parked the wrong way round, facing a wall of a leylandii and a dense bank of cotoneaster in a corner of the car park at the nursing home.

I was struggling: dangerously so.

Part of half-term had been brutal.

In our usual way, we had found ways to relax and have fun, visiting friends in Somerset and driving down to Exeter to collect Ranjit's Christmas present, a second-hand Pashley tricycle. But that enjoyment had been curtailed by a further decline in Moosh's condition.

I had long since stopped trying to fathom how many incremental mini-steps in weakening a human being could experience, yet still be determinedly holding on to the life that remained in them. Interleaved between our travels, I had anxiously added as many extra visits to the nursing home as tiredness would allow.

Once we fully returned home, I found myself living in fear that each time I left Moosh it would be the last time, and that the next phone call from the home would be terminal.

On the Saturday, I had sat in silence watching Moosh sleep, having arrived to find her tiny husk propped in the corner of her wingback chair. It now dwarfed her. Her breathing was shallow, almost inaudible, and her dentures pushed to be free of her lips.

When her son-receptor finally caused her to surface, her first act was to scold me, but her voice was barely a breath, "You should have woken me! Have you been watching me sleep?"

"Someone has to be here to catch your teeth, when they fall out," I teased. "You needed to sleep, and you looked very peaceful, apart from those duelling dentures. How are you today?"

I was surprised to hear her concede, "Not good. I've been very tired and weak; I don't have a lot of energy."

"No marathons this weekend, then?" I joked.

"Very funny. Maybe not."

She tried to poke her tongue out at me, but dislodged her teeth instead.

"Seriously though, Ma," I began, gently helping her teeth back into place, "do I need to ask if the doctor can visit you again? I am worried. You are not recovering your strength in the way that we hoped."

"Then stop making me laugh!" she wheezed, "It's probably not good for me."

She took a few seconds to gather herself, before continuing, "No, I don't think so. They are looking after me very well and I am taking my medicine."

Seeing the faux surprise on my face and further gentle mockery bubbling to my lips, she raised her hand just far enough to stop me, "But can you do one thing for me?"

I swallowed my witticism about how ill she must feel to be a) voluntarily praising the staff and b) taking her medication as prescribed. Instead I asked what she needed.

"Take me to Mass."

Seeing that her request had floored me, she added, "I'd be very grateful."

Her pleading was simply unfair and unrefusable pressure.

A part of me quailed, part of me stared in stunned disbelief, while a diminutive part of my brain began to problem solve.

Moosh asking to go to Church suggested to me that she yearned to feel even closer to God than her daily prayers brought her; her arthritic fingers kneading the rosary beads from the links of their chain were no longer affording her the solace that she sought. Although she hadn't asked me to call Father Guy to administer The Last Rites, I took her spiritual need as an indicator that she wanted to prepare against the possibility of dying. I knew that she trusted that I was fully versed in the absolute importance of ensuring that she received Extreme Unction, when the time came, but I guessed that she wanted to have every possible base covered.

Looking across at her diminished form, the challenge and risk of getting her safely to and from Church beggared me: she could barely sit up, in fact the chair was holding her up, and I was convinced that, if I attempted to move her, her already pitifully weak breathing would simply cease.

In the manager part of my brain, I was reasonably certain that there was no sensible, allowable risk assessment that would permit me to take Moosh to Church. The problem-solving son part of my brain was urging me to wrap her in layers of clothing and blankets, strap her in her wheelchair and risk the health repercussions.

"Let me ponder, Ma," I suggested and, by way of diversion, asked, "Are you strong enough for a game of Scrabble?"

"Always," she answered, but it was a lie.

That game brought one of my saddest moments with Moosh.

She desperately wanted to do our thing: Scrabble. It was what we did together in a world that had shrunk to the dimensions of her room. Usually, it brought her hours of shared time with me and, ordinarily, there were giggles-a-plenty as I caught her cheating, or amused her with my array of newly discovered rude words, or just reused old ones.

On that Saturday, try as she might, it was beyond her. She could not take tiles from the bag, nor place them on her rack, so I placed them for her. She could not build a word on the board without knocking out of place the tiles that had already been played. Cruellest of all, she could not think the words, but she tried.

Close to the end of a game in which I probably took every one of her goes for her, she insisted that she was making her own word. I already knew her hand, having placed the letters on her rack, but she was staring at her tiles and attempting to move them back and forth, toppling them and laboriously endeavouring to put them back, but unable to do so.

385

Frustrated to the point of tears, she mouthed, "I can't find an *E*."

Intrigued, I turned her rack towards me to see her hand, asking what word she wanted to put down. She had:

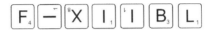

"FIDGET, but I can't find an *E*," she mumble-muttered, plaintively.

It is the most miniscule of tiny things that Moosh could not make a word in a board game, and that she could not see that she had only two of the letters required, or recognise that her letters were not oriented correctly with one *I* on its side, but the look of lost confusion on her face broke my heart: without our games of Scrabble and the love invested in them, what else could I give her?

"Shall we put FIX instead?" I suggested, Coldplay playing in my head.

At her weary nod, I placed her tiles for her, thinking to myself how apt my word choice was, however, not even the very respectable thirty-five points scored could prevent her from wilting further.

I finished the game, helping Moosh with the last couple of hands. She always hated the letter *I* and was inundated with them, but we (I) managed to use them all up and I packed away.

"I'm sorry I was so useless," Moosh said, attempting levity. "I used to be good at Scrabble, didn't I? I taught you everything you know Big Head."

I could not find the lightness required to respond with humour, so simply held her hand, submitting to the discomfort

386

of her writhing, gnarly grip. Surfacing from where I bury it, in my sub-conscience, was the fact that it was the twenty-fourth anniversary of Dad's death, and I was unwillingly pondering the coincidence of losing Moosh at the same time of year.

"It is so hard," she sighed, "feeling weak and useless on the outside. On the inside I can still run."

It was the closest I ever heard her come to self-pitying in a life that had given her so many valid excuses to be so. If I had not already decided to take her to Mass the next day, that cemented my resolve and made the solution very simple.

Later, having stayed longer than usual because I was worried that this would be the last time I left her, I told the staff that I wanted to bring Moosh to our house the next day and would come for her in the morning.

The next day, Sunday, I collected Moosh.

She had already been dressed against the cold by the staff, but I covered her in multiple blankets. At the car, I physically hauled her light but unable-to-help weight into the passenger seat and stowed her wheelchair in the boot. At the Oratory, I replicated the process in reverse to wheel her in to Church.

I have to confess to grinding my teeth through the entire service and especially the sermon, railing at a God that I no longer talked to for abandoning this woman, who talked to him constantly, but I still trundled her to the altar rail to receive communion and, despite myself, was touched by the delicacy with which the priest placed the host in her hand and the slightly longer moment for which he stood before her in benediction. I do understand the strength that Moosh drew from being in Church, having once upon a time shared her faith, and, although I no longer believed as she did, I was heartened that I had brought her back to the congregation that was so important to her.

Before going back to the nursing home, I took Moosh to our house. I did not tell Ranjit or the children how anxious I was, nor that I wanted them to have a chance to see her and make a fuss of her and hug her, should my fears be realised. It was obvious to anyone that she was weak, but going to Mass had brought about a small uplift, which was a good way for them to see her.

Having deposited her safely back in her room and assuring her, despite my fearfulness, that I would see her again on Tuesday, I took my leave of Moosh, carrying my mounting but unspoken apprehension with me.

And so it was that I found myself sat in my car, parked the wrong way round, because I had needed to take the wheelchair from the boot.

I found myself staring at the rich blanket of cotoneaster covered in vibrant orange-red berries, against a dense background of leylandii that blocked out any further view.

Entirely unbidden, I was overcome with a desperate desire to die.

I recognised that I was already feeling bereaved by a death that I felt was imminent. Added to this was the fact that I felt, should she survive, Moosh needed more time than I could afford to give. I knew that no one would judge me unkindly, if I said that I needed time away from work to be with her, but how much time? I knew also that school needed me: we had begun to be scrutinised and pressurised over pupil attainment results and there were multiple issues to deal with that I felt were my responsibility and should not be delegated. Most of all, I was crushed, not by Moosh's looming death, but by the loss of who she was: the fact that she was alive but that her quality of life was so wretched, and she was stoically accepting it. I swore to myself that I would never have an ending like hers.

I had never felt suicidal. Never.

However, on that Sunday afternoon, the weight of the entirely unexpected urge was crushingly overwhelming. My horizons drew in to just the blurring berries in front of me and I felt both helpless and hopeless and acknowledged a desperate wish to be free of the burdens and sadness of life. I expected a panic attack to overtake me, but none came. Instead, I simply sat, inert, too scared to move, in case by doing so, I should act upon the impulse. The storm of emotion inside my head was entirely new to me: the grief, the need to escape, the calculating of ways out, the sense of guilt for even considering leaving my family behind.

Ultimately, I managed to calm myself and turn the ignition, reversing away from the cotoneaster and driving home with methodical care. I remember, vividly, indicating right to turn into the flow of traffic, forcing myself to breathe and to concentrate, checking each manoeuvre, as if in slow motion.

Once home, I was too scared to tell Ranjit how I was feeling and, possibly foolishly, did not tell anyone else, but forced myself to focus intently on being present for her and the children.

I returned to school the next day and, stunningly, Moosh rallied.

But neither of our alarms were over.

52

Heaven

Moosh's rally, after going to Mass, continued in the weeks that followed.

Clearly she was never going to regain the ability to run, or even walk around unaided, or to mount any final, serious escape bid, but she was returning to the former self that the staff recognised; the independent terror who wilfully ignored all entreaties to countenance risk assessments.

For me, this meant that our weekends returned to their norm of passing companionable time watching TV, skimming newspapers and magazines, playing Scrabble and sharing videos of Her Most Wonderfulness on her trike, gliding along serenely, seemingly far too posh to pedal, (but in truth rolling down a gentle incline).

Moosh was very taken by the idea of HMW swanning down the cycle lanes of the Languedoc on her tricycle, either heading along the Canal du Midi to search out a spot for aperitifs, or with the parcel shelf laden with a hamper to be enjoyed at the beach. She saw the possibilities of a jaunty freedom in that Pashley, which brought on recollections of gadding around Malaya in her MG with her beloved Fury.

I revelled in the image of her speeding along, vibrantly alive, in her sports car with a German Shepherd in the passenger seat, its mouth grinning and tongue lolling, but could not help reminding her of our one and only abortive attempt to get her driving during my lifetime. Initially, she looked abashed at the remembered failure, but soon we were both guffawing our loudest at the memory of her claiming that modern cars were not up to the standard of vintage ones: on Black Rock Sands in Snowdonia, she had been utterly unable to master clutch and gears, so we had made do with her hiccupping my Vauxhall Nova across the beach in first, more stalling than travelling.

As November progressed, I was stunned that she had a point of view on the contestants of *I'm A Celebrity . . .Get Me Out Of Here*, throwing her loyalties behind the veteran jockey, Willie Carson, and predicting with utter confidence that he was sure to win.

When I commented on how impressed I was that she was staying up to watch, she hooted that of course she was not actually watching it, it being on at the time that she liked to pray. Not watching did not prevent her from holding some very strong, newspaper-fuelled opinions, and her prayerfulness did not diminish the acid tang of her comments about several of the female contestants.

Her backing of Willie harked back to being enamoured of him as one of the captains on *A Question Of Sport*; a crush of almost 30 years. When I pointed out that this prolonged length of swoon was longer than my Dad enjoyed, she pouted, although it is not possible to pout properly with false teeth.

It was a joy to see her cognitive abilities return alongside her sense of humour. It should not mean so much, but it was a relief that she was able to get back to playing her own hand in Scrabble and to fake glower at me, when I put down *yoni* for maybe the hundredth time in our lifetime of playing. I mocked her affectionately that she could take the moral high ground on my choice of Scrabble words, but be uncharitably scathing about contestants on a TV show.

She was very aware of her recovery and of how concerned we had been. A part of her was anxious too. Her episode of intense weakness and her need to attend Mass, resulted in a conversation that held enormous significance for her.

We had talked over the papers and magazines, tidied away the Scrabble and scorepad and I was gathering together laundry, making ready to leave, when Moosh asked, "Can I talk to you about something?"

Sensing a seriousness in her tone, I resisted the temptation to make light of the moment and opted for sitting back down and saying, "Of course, what is it?"

She took a moment to gather herself and then blurted out, "I am worried about what will happen when I die."

Misunderstanding, I tried to reassure her, "Ma, you've talked with Alyson and been very clear about what you want us to do."

Indeed, she had, having gone into the fine detail of her funeral plan and the different bequests that she wanted Neil and I to make on her behalf. It was all part of her still unwritten, but clearly understood, End of Life Plan.

"And I know that I didn't call Father Guy, last month," I continued, "but I know that I must arrange for the Last

Sacrament, when that moment comes. I won't forget. I promise."

She actually wrung her hands, shaking her head, "No, I mean *afterwards*, to me and you."

Initially perplexed, I waited for more, but as Moosh looked at me so imploringly, trying to find her words, my realisation first flickered, then sparked and I hesitantly filled the gap that she couldn't yet, "You are thinking about after you are gone?"

Her forlorn nod prompted me to continue, "You mean what will happen to you and I? Do you mean in a life after death way?"

She nodded again, looking bereft, and mouthed, "We won't see each other, will we?"

Understanding having fully dawned, I moved round to hug her, as fiercely as I dared.

This was a conversation a long time in the delaying and one that I would have happily swerved, if at all possible.

"Well, you'll be in Heaven, won't you? Well, unless you keep being bitchy about those poor women on *I'm A Celebrity*."

She managed a chuckle, "I hope so," before adding solemnly, "I pray so."

"Ma, seriously," I couldn't stop myself from trying to keep the conversation light, "you pray more than Mother Teresa! I'm sure that God hears you and mutters, 'Geraldine, you again?' You've had The Last Rites enough times to make me think that you are at least half cat. I know that you can't get to confession at Church, but I bet that you proclaim your acts of contrition from this chair and that God listens. And, let's face it, you can't get up to too much badness in here.

393

Although, you'd better make sure that you keep treating the staff nicely or else there will be no Christmas presents and no Heaven."

I just could not resist that last little reminder to maintain goodwill to all, including the staff.

She nudged me with a pointy elbow and said what I now knew was on her mind, "But you won't join me there, will you?"

And there it was, with a silent but percussive *boom*: her dread and her judgement, "How can you come to somewhere you do not believe in?"

Moosh feared for my mortal soul. To her, I was a lost non-believer, her son who she had hoped might become a Catholic priest, but who had turned away from a budding, but nevertheless deeply held vocation, and who had, for many years, been searching along different spiritual paths, none of which, as yet, had reached any solid conclusions.

At her most unreasonable, she blamed Ranjit for this wayward straying, as she had at the stunning Tropen Museum in Amsterdam.

I had been wandering, agog, between statues of Buddha and Shiva, when Moosh scurried through the gallery, her eyes fixed firmly on the floor, asserting vehemently to Ranjit, "He wasn't interested in these dark religions until *you* came along."

Although she did eventually forgive Ranjit for not being the good Catholic (preferably Irish) girl that she had hoped I would marry, she could never quite forgive me for my spiritual deviation from the way she had brought me up, a faith that had served her so well.

Moreover, she knew that my beliefs about life after death

jarred entirely with hers. She believed absolutely in living a life worthy of a place in Heaven, and had striven for as long as she could remember to secure salvation. It grieved her that I had chosen not to follow her belief in Heaven. As she faced her own death, this had transformed into her anxiety that we would never see one another again.

So, I tried, however clumsily, to staunch her fear, opening with, "Ma, I know that we have very different beliefs about God."

That was an understatement: I veered from outright atheism, to a searching agnosticism, to my own individual construct that matches my spirituality, but I now needed to find a way to put her at ease, while being honest to myself.

"For you, God is something outside of you, who you are answerable to. For me, we should not do things because we fear divine retribution, nor because we hope for a reward. For me, my idea of God is that voice inside us that enables us to choose the right way to treat people and is the sum total of all the acts of goodness that we perform in our lives. I don't want a reward, I just want to be able to look back on my life and feel sure that I treated people well. I'm not trying to get into Heaven - although Hell does sound scary.

"I know that seeing me in Heaven is important to you and that it comforts you that you will meet Daddy again, as long as he didn't mess up too badly.

"It may not help, but what I believe is that you will always be with me. As long as I live, your spirit will be inside me. As long as my children live, the love that you have shown them and the example that you have given them will shine through them. When Jess and Liam get married, your love will be there with us. Whenever I look at Harvey, I will remember how much you loved him just the way he is. Whenever I watch Alex play, I will know that you set him on his journey.

"The best that I can offer is that when I do woodwork with Dad's tools, I can feel him near me, watching me, guiding me. When I talk to Alex and Arun about fatherhood, I have Dad's voice in my ear, beseeching me to be a better father than he judged himself to be; I encourage them with him in my heart.

"And so it will be with you. When I teach children at school to question the way people in the world are treated, I will be speaking your truth. I will tell them that you taught me to question the genocide of the native peoples of the Americas and the oppression of black people in South Africa, before it was accepted to think your way. Whenever I teach girls to expect to be treated with respect and boys to treat them with respect, and that women and men are different, but equal, I will remember that you taught me that, when it was not the prevalent view.

"I can not say that I will join you in Heaven, because that would be pretty hypocritical of me, but you have always taught me to try to live a good life in the way that Jesus taught. What about all of the people, who are brought up from birth in other religions, who never had a choice about their faith, like Jews and Sikhs and Muslims? If they live their lives well, won't they have a good chance of getting into Paradise or Heaven? What about a Native North American or an Inuit Eskimo? If they live a good life, but have never been Christian, are they barred from Heaven?"

I saw a gestalt light of hope ignite in her eyes, as my fragments of thought coalesced for her, and so pressed my advantage, "I've always tried to live my life well. I have

Christian friends who say that I am a good Christian, and Sikh friends who say I would make a passable Sikh, and Muslim friends who say I would make a good Muslim. I know it sounds like boasting, but I must be doing something right."

She was smiling and nodding, so I closed by saying, hopefully, "What if I keep trying to live my life well? Maybe then you can say to Saint Peter, 'He did try to follow Jesus's example, even if he got a bit lost.' I might just make it, mightn't I?"

And that was enough.

It was not a theological dissertation that would stand up to close scrutiny, but at that moment, for Moosh, it soothed her, and it was my truth.

For myself, I was still reeling from the strength of the impulse to end my life.

I had no idea where the thought had come from. I had not acted upon it and I was relieved that, although I kept reflecting on the episode in the car park and trying to unpick it, I was controlling the urge and, rightly or wrongly, keeping it to myself.

It would have traumatised Moosh, had she even the slightest inkling that I had contemplated testing Saint Peter's judgement, even before he had a chance to welcome her.

VI

Part Six

Taking Flight
February 2012

53

Not Quite La Dolce Vita

For Her Most Wonderfulness and I, a favourite relaxation is to travel; whether near or far, just being away has always been our diversion from the demands of life. As we moved into 2012, we both knew that we needed some time away.

Crucially, we had Moosh's fervent blessing, because of where we chose to go.

We love to go on European city breaks. Our list of places we hope to visit is long, but so far we have visited just a few: Paris, Amsterdam, Koln, Barcelona, Seville and Venice.

Despite being born in a village in the Punjab, HMW loves the bright lights and bustle of big, vibrant cities. She loves, even more, the whole game of researching the top, must-see attractions, happily trawling for hours through the guidebooks of Michelin, Lonely Planet, Rough Guide and Dorling Kindersley to create itineraries, making sure that we pack in as many must-sees as possible into the time that we've got.

The only things that top the ticking off and critiquing of

all the major sites, are:

a) to do everything for the best bargain price possible

b) to "discover" somewhere that we had not initially considered, such as Venice's Jewish ghetto or the oldest candle shop in Barcelona.

Theoretically, these trips are a time to be together, away from the pressures of work and sharing some "us" time, but don't be getting any wrong ideas, there is nothing remotely romantic about this "us" time, none of that. By the end of each day of metro/tram/bus jumping and trooping around a city, our legs are aching, bloody stumps and all we can do is to competitively share our photos and agree that hers are the best – every time.

So, in February half-term, we headed to Rome for HMW's version of *la dolce vita*.

She was characteristically prepared, armed with a list of Ancient Roman sites, museums and churches that we must visit, affordable places to eat and details of tourist deals to allow us access to several attractions at reduced rates and to eat affordably. We were both ready for the break of being away from home, the diversion of experiencing Rome together.

I was looking forward to sharing with HMW my fond recollections of a couple of days spent in the city, as an eighteen-year-old, with a group of school friends. We had convinced Fr. Round, the master who taught Ancient Studies, to take us to the beaches of France and Italy under the cunning guise of suggesting a historical tour as a school trip. He had willingly agreed (to the tour, not the beaches) and so off we had pootled down through France, via the

Roman sites in Lyon and Orange and the Pont du Gard, before we nonchalantly threw in the request to visit Frejus, on the Cote d'Azur. We judged that suggesting Saint-Tropez would be way too obvious a ploy.

Much to our youthful, testosterone-fuelled dismay, our thinly veiled plot to lounge on the topless beaches were thwarted by a thunderstorm of biblical proportions on our very first (and, as it turned out, only) night, which flattened every last one of our tents, while we were out on the town, being laddish. Almost certainly aware that our devastation was not entirely for our tents, Fr. Round jovially bundled us and our sodden tents into our minibus and drove us through the night, almost 500 miles, to Rome.

I have wonderful memories of arriving in the Eternal City, very, very early one bright July morning, with Fr. Round driving our minibus around all the major sites, utterly devoid of tourists and so free of traffic that he cavalierly scooted the wrong way up one-way streets. Ever an animated man, Fr. Round became even more effusive, as he shared the city where he had trained and which he clearly loved, all done at the best breakneck speed that a pretty knackered minibus could muster. Before HMW and I embarked on our trip, I spent a happy hour looking back through my photo albums of that youthful trip and found a picture of Fr. Round posing, orator-like, beneath a statue of a Roman dignitary. He was a lovely man.

Moosh was almost more excited than us, thinking Rome was a great idea.

I was worried about leaving her, but had arranged for each of the children to visit her, so she would have many more than her normal quota of visitors. Despite the burgeoning catalogue of hurt, Aly was once again on call, if there was any drama, and hoped to drive down for a couple of days, if life in Loftus allowed.

Moosh was delighted that we were planning to go to the Vatican, one of her favourite places on Earth, and we had compared notes from our respective visits. She was certain that I would see the Pope, which I suggested was unlikely, and she hoped that I would attend Mass, which I warned her was equally unlikely. I did, however, promise to say a prayer for her at St. Peter's.

Her Most Wonderfulness and I did it all, or at least most of it.

We immersed ourselves in *Roma*'s riches: the Colosseum, the Forum, the Palatine Hill, Piazza Navona, the Pantheon, the Trevi Fountain and St. Peter's Square. We got up early and went to bed late to try to fit everything in. We yomped to the Roman Steps after dark to tick it off HMW's list, only for her to declare that, like the Colosseum, they are over-rated – whisper it quietly, but according to her the Colosseum, probably Rome's most iconic landmark, is 'rather run down and not a patch on the amphitheatre in Nimes'. Everywhere, even the Colosseum, was captured in our amateurish photographs, with each of us trying to outdo the other.

We took the Bus Tour to make sure that we had seen as much of everything as humanly possible. I'm not the greatest fan of bus tours, ever since the humiliation of *Barcelona Bottom*, when I was followed through Gaudi's city one sticky July, by a cacophonously cackling HMW, who was in hysterics at the site of my drenched shorts hanging from my traumatised buttocks, soaked by the sweat generated through sitting on an unforgiving hard, plastic seat on a sweltering day. That being said, I have to admit that Rome's Bus Tour (in a far from *scorchio* February) served us very well.

If the guidebooks are correct, and I am sure they must be, there are over 365 churches in Rome, more than one for every day of the year. Slightly bizarrely for a Sikh by birth and an ultra-lapsed Catholic, on our city breaks, we always visit the churches and cathedrals. We visit other holy sites, but always churches. In Rome we visited dozens of churches, not hundreds, but so very many. We hardly passed one without popping in: I have the photos, oodles of them. We didn't quite manage to light a votive candle for Moosh in every single one, but enough to illuminate a small town.

We saved the big one for last: Saint Peter's Basilica.

My entirely justified reservation about bus tours did not prevent me from being more than a little dismayed by HMW's announcement, after using the perfectly effective and comfortable bus, that Rome is in fact a very small city, or at least the touristy centre is, and so, for our visit to the Vatican, we could easily walk there and back. However, my dismay counted for nothing, because HMW, on her tour guide setting, would give Mussolini a run for his money in the dictatorship stakes. So off we set. I would never tell her, but it was a fabulous walk that took me back to Fr. Round's whirlwind tour, albeit at the rather slower, non-motorised, pace of a forced march, punctuated by photo stops.

Before visiting the basilica itself, we gawped through

the Sistine Chapel, marvelling at Renaissance frescos by Botticelli and his contemporaries, and craning upwards to gaze at Michelangelo's wondrous ceiling, especially *The Creation of Adam*.

Having lulled me into open-mouthed amazement, HMW played her absolute Top Trump Roman Must See: Rome from the top of St. Peter's dome. Getting to the top of the cupola is described by delightfullyitaly.com as: "a great opportunity to enjoy a fantastic and dizzying city panorama"- *dizzying* being the key word. She played this card in the clear knowledge that I struggle horribly with vertigo and confined spaces. After the lift, which cuts out 320 steps, there are still 231 to go, inside the ever narrowing, curved slope of the dome.

All my, frankly unadmirable, wheedling about heights and claustrophobia were quashed with, "Geraldine will love to see the pictures we take from the top. You won't get views like that from anywhere else."

She should write her own tourist guidebook (AND one on how to waltz through life getting your own way). But, I have to admit (ever so quietly) that the photographs of the statues of the apostles *and* of St. Peter's Square *and* the Vatican Gardens *and* down into the basilica were all stunning.

Despite my spiritual movement away from formal religion in general and Roman Catholicism in particular, there are church experiences and sacred spaces that simply fill me with awe and tug at my lost vocation. The quality of light in Paddy's Wigwam in Liverpool once moved me to unexpected tears, so too the stunning architecture in Gaudi's Sagrada Familia and, within it, Subirach's sublime bronze Lord's Prayer door, featuring fifty languages. On a far less grand

scale, the tiny, but beautifully painted Chapel of Notre-Dam
e-de-la-Salette on top of Mont Saint-Clair in Sete, has much
the same effect and I can sit there, lost in reverie, for hours .

With *The Pieta* and St. Peter's Tomb, Saint Peter's Basilica,
hub of the Roman Catholic religion, is jaw dropping, but
since my first visit as an eighteen year old, it is Bernini's *Dove
of the Holy Spirit* that has stayed with me: just seeing it in
my mind's eye fills me with wonder and a longing for the
spiritual certainty that has eluded me. After years together,
HMW is finely attuned to this yearning in me and always
drifts off to allow me to dwell and wallow in my loss of faith.

That day in the basilica, as HMW explored, wide eyed, I sat
staring at the dove haloed in golds and ambers, and found
myself reflecting on the fact that it is one of the only images
of faith that was special to both Moosh and I. I knew that
she would be delighted to hear that I had sat in reverent awe
beneath it. I could picture her sitting in exactly the same pose
as mine, her face suffused with a very similar expression.

In that moment, I felt myself washed by a warm wave
of closeness with her and affectionate admiration of the
strength that kept her battling, knowing that, despite the
uncertainties of my own faith, it was her spiritual certainty
that underpinned her fortitude. And I was grateful and
uplifted.

The positivity, however, was fleeting, followed instantly by
a forceful counter current of sadness at Moosh's frailty and
her sense of being betrayed by a body that she willed to do
God's bidding. Witnessing her forbearance was too painful
for us and I did not know how much more she herself could
endure, or should be expected to by God.

Emotionally torn by, on the one hand, the sensation of

spiritual connection with Moosh through 'our' dove and, on the other, a morose fear of impending loss, I sought to avert the sadness that I was struggling to hold at bay by taking more photos for Moosh, and then I went in search of somewhere to pray.

In such a wondrous church, full of pilgrims and visitors and tongues from across the globe, it can be difficult to find quietness, but the Blessed Sacrament Chapel is set aside for silent prayer. I entered, conflicted. I had not prayed on a personal level for decades. As headteacher at our school of many faiths, when I led the children in prayer, our prayer primarily took the form of thoughtful reflection on our life paths and sharing sincere thankfulness, rather than entreaties to God or giving praise.

Yet, here I was, kneeling down knowing that I was in need, not quite talking to God, but nakedly facing up to my feelings and speaking them in my mind, desperate.

When I emerged, Ranjit, having already lit a candle for Mum, squeezed my hand and suggested that we go to the gift shop. She knew that I would buy a crucifix. Moosh loved crucifixes and, over the years, I had bought her a collection of them. I always found it easy to find the right one and was quickly pleased with myself.

I was surprised to see that Ranjit also clutched a small package. A little shyly, she showed me a Pope John Paul II prayer book and a bookmark in the form of a prayer card.

Tentatively, she said, "I thought Geraldine would like these. Do you think they will be OK?"

My eyes filled.

54

El Papa's Prayer Book

We flew home from Rome on the Friday at the end of our half-term week, exhausted but refreshed and ready for whatever life threw at us. It was five years to the week, since we had collected Moosh from Loftus.

The last thing I did, before we headed for bed, was to transfer all of our photos to my laptop. This was not a straightforward job, as it entailed further competition over whose photo of each site and each viewpoint was the best. It also involved me cropping my photos (and some of HMW's, without her knowing) so that I was happy with them. Lastly, I collected together a folder of photos to show Moosh our trip without going through several hundred pictures – there were still over one hundred images set up ready for a slideshow.

Next morning, I bought the usual essentials (green bananas, Arrowroot biscuits, Bourneville, *Hello!* and *OK!*), plus a luxury Terry's Chocolate Orange and a precautionary bar of Pears and headed down to see Moosh, shopping in one hand and laptop bag in the other. I was so excited to share

Rome with her that I would have bounded into her room, but I chose instead to sneak my head round the door.

She was sitting there, expectant and perky.

"I've been waiting. I knew you'd come early," she beamed.

Her hug was a crusher, little bony arms creating a vice-like grip, until my back wouldn't allow me to lean down any longer.

She released most of me, but held my forearms and said, "I've missed you."

"I've missed you a bit; just a tiny bit," I grinned, retrieving her glasses, which had been dislodged in her power hug, "but Rome was fab. My God, your glasses are filthy. I'll give them a clean, because you are going to need them."

She blitzed me with a torrent of eager questions: "What was it like? Was the weather good? It snowed when the rugby was on, didn't it? Did you like the Vatican?"

"It was amazing. Just what we needed. Rome's smaller than I remember, but packed with so much to do. We couldn't fit everything in. We'll have to go back. You're right, it had snowed and we saw fields and mountains covered as we flew in, but most of the snow had gone in Rome itself. I've brought photos on my laptop. Does that answer all of your questions?"

"I knew you'd love going back. Did Ranjit like it too? Did she like the Vatican?"

"She loved Rome. She marched us everywhere. I've renamed her Benitojit. She made me walk miles."

"What did she think of St. Peter's?"

"We couldn't go. She didn't feel up to it. We'd left it to the last day, but we needed to rest."

Moosh's face clouded, but she rallied on her best behaviour

410

with, "Poor thing. I know she'd have liked it. You'll just have to take her back."

"So I can turn her into a good Catholic girl?" I teased.

"Because she likes churches and I know she'd like it."

She was trying to conceal her let down feeling.

"Shall I thrash you at Scrabble first? Or would you like to see our photos first? I've made a little slideshow for you, so that I can show you where we went. You can see which bits you remember. Do you think you'll remember any?"

The last question brought a firm pinch.

"Rome first. Then Scrabble. Two games. Do you want some chocolate orange? Do you need the telly socket?" she fired, the last vestiges of disappointment retreating.

"The laptop's all charged for you. You can stare at photos for hours. Two games, if we've got time, but I need to do a bit of schoolwork this afternoon. The chocolate is for you. I'm trying not to," I answered, as I cleared her table, placed the laptop in front of her and powered up.

"You can just watch the slideshow, or you can click back and forwards with the mouse buttons."

"Mouse buttons!" she giggled. "Why are they called mouse buttons?"

"You always ask that. Do you remember how to use them?"

"I do. I don't forget things," she pretended to be affronted. "I'll click the mousey buttons."

And off we went on our e.trip, punctuated by Moosh's ooohs and aaahs and a stream of observations, recollections and questions: "Oooh, the Trevi Fountain. Isn't it fabulous? There weren't many people there, were there? The Roman Steps. Did you go to the top or just take photos? You went

411

at night?"

I waited for the slap. I knew there would be a slap. And, sure enough, here it came, a swipe on the arm.

"You said you didn't go to St. Peter's!"

Another swipe.

"That's just from the bus, Ma. We went on a bus tour that goes past it. Were there many people when you went? We'll go inside next time."

"You'll have to take her back."

Click. Click. Click.

"Which church is this? It's beautiful."

"I can't remember, Ma. There were lots of churches. So many churches!"

"Over three hundred and sixty-five!" she confirmed what our guidebooks had told us.

Click. Whack! A very hard slap.

"You did go!" she exclaimed delightedly.

"We did, Ma!"

I released the repressed laughter that had been building for the last dozen clicks. The anticipation was just like when you are playing Hide and Seek as a child, and you know the Seeker is getting close, and you are overcome by the need to wee. I needed a wee, but her delight was too great for me to leave.

"We went to the Sistine Chapel. That hands painting is amazing in real life, isn't it? And we climbed right to the top of the cupola. I hated it, but the view is mega, look. And *The Pieta* was even more striking than I remembered, soulful and poignant. And I sat and stared at our dove for ages; it's just so stunning and awe inspiring, isn't it? The colours were amazing. I felt very close to you."

412

She squeezed my hand in her knobbly, arthritic way until the rotation made my hand uncomfortable, but I did not pull away, and she beamed, wordlessly radiant.

"I brought some things for you. Would you like them now?"

She nodded, still beaming, still silent.

First, I gave her my crucifix. She studied it and held it to her chest, her eyes clouding again, but happily this time.

She looked at her line of crucifixes and I said, "Shall I hang it up? I even brought a nail!"

She nodded and I handed her Ranjit's envelope, saying, "Ranjit chose this for you."

Delicately, almost reverentially, as if she knew what it contained, Moosh accepted the envelope, opened it and slipped out the prayer book and prayer card.

She looked up at me with pleasure blossoming on her face and asked, "Ranjit chose these?"

"She did," I answered. "You might make a good Catholic girl out of her yet!"

She grinned and said, "Oh, no. I don't need to. She's very special, just as she is. I should tell her that, shouldn't I?"

She paused, caught in that emotion, while inside I danced elatedly, celebrating her admission of Ranjit's worth, before she continued reverently, "He'll be a saint soon, do you think? Such a lovely man. I'll read this later."

"You can read it now, but it will mean less Scrabble. Your choice." I challenged.

I thrashed her at Scrabble. Twice. There was only minor cheating, two hidden *E*s and some help to create QUIETEN on a triple word score, but she concentrated well and didn't invent any new words. All the words she conjured were relatable to the tiles on her letter holder. I scored over 400 in each game, so we were both happy.

Before I packed up to leave, I asked, "Would you like me to leave the laptop with you, so that you can look through the pictures again? The battery will last for a few hours. I can collect it on Tuesday."

"No. Bring it next week and we can look at them together. I don't want it stolen."

"No one will steal it, Ma. You know that. But I will bring it back."

I quietened and hesitated before saying, "I prayed, Ma. At St. Peter's. I prayed for you."

She cocked her head, slightly surprised, but more delighted, "What did you pray for?"

I held her hands and whispered, "It probably wasn't a very good prayer, Ma. I'm very out of practice. But I asked that you find peace. Was that OK?"

My voice cracked and we both misted over.

When we regained our composure, Moosh said, "It's a good prayer, Alistair. Thank you."

As I was hugging her to leave, she said, "Please thank Ranjit for my prayer book. Tell her I'll treasure it."

I did my thing of leaving and sneaking back, leaving and sneaking back, leaving and sneaking back and she was laughing and shooing me out, giggling, "Go now!"

She was already opening Ranjit's book.

55

The Big Call

The Sunday after Rome was a sofa day: a day for holding off
the world ahead of the second half of the school year; a day
for rest.

By the simple law of the calendar, the six Sundays at the end
of each school holiday are, unavoidably, the day before the
start of a new half-term. Consequently, those are rarely ever
my favourite days. It is not that I do not enjoy being at school;
I do. Once I am there, I willingly throw myself in and love it.
However, on those Sundays, I always feel the beginnings of
the renewed build-up of pressure, mentally reviewing the
state of play and plotting the way ahead - whatever vessel it
is that I have just spent the entire holiday voiding of stress, is
slowly allowing the first grains of the weight of responsibility
and accountability to trickle back in.

On that particular Sunday, half of the school year gone,
there were five months more to go and I could physically feel
the external pressure building on us as a school. We were
still being notified that we were vulnerable, because our data

see-sawed, dependent on the emotional needs of each cohort, and we were being told that we must be more consistent. We were striving to get our heads around a new curriculum demand that our youngest children must learn phonics to an arbitrary standard. Many could not yet speak English, but we had to teach them letter sounds and word building and how to decipher nonsense words. Before Ranjit woke, I made time to go through my diary to check the demands of the week and term ahead: for me the act of checking was quite routine, just the beginning of pressure.

The cocktail of Moosh's declining health and demands of work meant that it had been important for Ranjit and me to get away for that few days of relaxation during the week, but the excitement of travelling and exploring always carries the backwash of tiredness. So, once Ranjit emerged from our room, I hid all signs of work and we had an undemanding morning of television and catch up phone calls sharing our Roman highlights, followed by a lazy lunch and plans to maybe watch football or a film in the afternoon. It was a day for dressing gowns and duvets and gently accepting that tomorrow we would be back at school.

When I answered the phone, I assumed that it was another of Ranjit's girlfriends calling for a Rome catch up and to share news.

"Mark, it is Sylvia from the nursing home. I am ringing about Geraldine."

There was a different quality to her voice; a new one that immediately arrested me. It was beyond her usual professionalism.

"She collapsed in her room and we judged that she needed

416

an ambulance. She has been taken to City Hospital. Can you go to join her? She will be in A&E."

Responding to her tone, I shifted rapidly through the gears from carefully curated gentle repose, to concerned alertness, then to decisively responsive, answering, "I can be there in about twenty minutes. Do I need to collect anything for her?"

Sylvia's answer was succinct, "Mark this does not look like a fall. Geraldine has collapsed. Don't come here on your way. Go straight to the hospital. You might want to call your sister. She may want to come."

"Is that where we are?" I checked. "Does Alyson need to come?"

Given the gravity of Sylvia's warning, I readied myself with remarkable calm, shaving and dressing neatly, because I have always been convinced that the way that you present yourself in challenging situations can have a bearing on the way you are treated.

As I drove, my brain occupied itself by recounting the many emergencies that had taken me around the corner of Sandon Road onto City Road: Arun's catalogue of football injuries; my own brush with Legionnaires Disease when Dr. Kay warned me against driving myself to hospital, as he was not 100% certain that I would survive to reach there; and the time that kidney stones caused me to scream for almost the entire journey, panicking our friend Steve, who had been called on to drive me.

As I continued down City Road, in highly sensitised slow motion, I noted changes to the cityscape since I had last taken any notice of a road that I travelled so regularly. Turning off Dudley Road into the hospital, I congratulated myself on having had the presence of mind to check that I had sufficient money to pay for car parking, however long I needed to stay. Parked, paid and displayed, I checked the charge on my mobile phone, telling myself that I would call Aly, once I had information from the staff in A&E.

It was only as I walked from the car that I consciously focussed on Moosh and Sylvia's warning tone and steeled myself.

I was shown through to the Medical Assessment Unit.

There was no waiting. I was met with care and support and taken into a curtained cubicle. Relief washed over me at the sight of Moosh moving. Her dyskinesia was the clearest sign of life. More than that, her eyes were open, and she was moving her head to look around the room. I realised that I had been guarding against the expectation that I would not find her alive.

The young nurse told me that a doctor would arrive shortly to apprise me of what had happened and what would happen next and then she left me to be with Moosh, telling me to call if I needed anything.

Once we were alone, I looked down at Moosh and held her hand. She was diminutive but her hand gripped mine. Her eyes scanned the space above her, unfocussed.

"I'm here, Ma," I whispered. "How are you?"

I am not certain that I expected a verbal response, but Moosh did not answer. Her grasp on my hand continued, but her eyes seemed to be simultaneously seeking yet vacant. I positioned myself so that my face was directly above her at arm's length, but ensuring that I was visible and recognisable.

Accepting that Moosh was not able to answer me, I applied my knowledge gleaned from countless hospital dramas: "Talk to her – the sound of your voice will reassure her/let her know that you are here/bring her back. Keep talking."

I am unable to recall my exact words, but I can still vividly see myself with Moosh's hand in mine, keeping up a steady monologue, probably of inconsequential musings. What I do remember starkly is the concern that grew in me that Moosh was not seeing me, despite her eyes ranging around the cubicle, and not appearing to hear me, even when I bowed my lips to her ear. There was no flicker of her registering my presence, but I kept up my unrelenting, one-sided conversation, until a doctor joined me.

Without registering his name or waiting for him to speak, I shared my fear with him, "Doctor, is my Mum seeing me? She is looking around the room, but I do not think that she can focus on me. I have tried speaking to her, but all that she is able to do is hold on to my hand."

With utmost care and gentleness, he informed me that Moosh had suffered a bleed in her brain and that her position was precarious. He advised that I should let family members know. He explained that, should Moosh survive, the likelihood was that significant brain damage had occurred. With genuine tenderness he added that Moosh was not seeing me and that, although her hand was holding mine, this was almost certainly a result of her dyskinetic movement appearing to be a grip, rather than a conscious action.

Processing his words, I managed to say, "Doctor, my mother's faith is very important to her. She is a Roman Catholic. She has instructed me to arrange for The Last

Rites, if she is at risk of dying. Is it time for me to do that?"

"I think that would be best, Mark," he confirmed kindly. "Please invite the priest to come to your mother, here. We will not move her until he has been."

Sitting next to Moosh, as if needing her to witness me fulfilling her foremost wish, I called the Oratory.

56

Taking Flight

Having sent me on ahead to reach Moosh as soon as possible, Ranjit arrived, after organising everything at home.

We would soon celebrate our silver wedding anniversary and had been one another's closest friend for most of the last thirty years.

All marriages are unique. Ours is typified by laughter (often at one another's expense) and a strong willingness to butt heads over our points of view, sometimes heatedly. We will revisit issues many times and there are bones of contention that are woven into the fabric of our relationship, ornamenting it like decorative beads braided into hair. We can sustain a hurt for days and can appear fiery, but our arguing is based on a deep respect for the other and a determination to find our truth. However, when confronted by any challenge in our lives, our support for one another is unswerving and unstinting.

In my entire life, I have never been more grateful for Ranjit's presence than on that afternoon and into the early evening.

It was brutal.

As I finished sharing the doctor's views and prognosis with Ranjit, Fr. Erasmus arrived in response to my phone call to the Oratory.

A tiny part of me was devastated that it was not Fr. Guy who would administer the Last Rites to Moosh for the final time, but Fr. Erasmus's open, friendly face and the sincerity of his compassion instantly mollified me.

Introductions made and the facts of Moosh's condition shared, I was taken aback by Fr. Erasmus's suggestion that Ranjit and I be present for the giving of the sacrament. My conscience compelled me to declare my spiritual ambivalence and crisis of faith and to add that for Ranjit, a Sikh by birth, the closest that she had come to Catholicism was attendance at Catholic primary and secondary schools and a Catholic teacher training college.

Fr. Erasmus laughed quietly, but with comforting warmth, before saying, "Mark, the sacrament is given to Geraldine, but it is for your comfort, also; for both of you, regardless of your beliefs."

It felt good to be laughing, however restrainedly, while readying to prepare Moosh for death in the way that she had repeatedly stipulated we should. It also felt right that a lapsed Sikh stood supportively on one side of an even more lapsed Catholic, while a priest stood on the other and carried out Moosh's most devoutly held requirement.

To add to my surprise, Fr. Erasmus invited us to participate in elements of the sacrament, including us rather than rendering us mute witnesses. I was entirely unprepared, but found myself strengthened for what was to come and reassured that Moosh would be gratified. Ranjit was also deeply affected by her inclusion.

I wish that I could say that Moosh registered the sacrament, or that it appeared to ease her, but that would be untrue. Moosh continued to writhe and her eyes cast around the space above her, unseeing. As Fr. Erasmus had predicted, the easing was in Ranjit and me.

Mirroring our earlier laughter, my verbal thanks to him were restrained, as I sought to bottle my emotions, but there was an impassioned strength in the clasp of my hand, as I shook his on his departure.

While waiting for Fr. Erasmus and Ranjit, I had rung Alyson to let her know what had happened and that, in likelihood, we were looking at hours rather than days. Neil made the difficult calculation that, while it was potentially possible to reach Moosh three hours after they set out, with the need to arrange care for Harvey and to get ready, it was unlikely that they would arrive in time to see Moosh alive. We agreed that, if the prognosis proved incorrect and Moosh survived the night, Aly would come down the following day.

Ranjit had explained to Arun and Ayesha the gravity of the situation we were facing. Neither of us wanted the two of them to experience what we feared we might face over the coming hours and so had not asked whether they wanted to come to the hospital, nor invited them to do so.

Alex was at university and, in my brain, had left home. He was the same age as I had been when Ranjit and I bought our first house and a year short of the age I was when we had married; in short, he was an adult to be informed of what was happening and consulted as to whether he wanted to travel in an attempt to say his farewells to his grandmother. At that point in his life, Moosh was almost certainly the most powerful influence he had ever had. I was silently relieved when he concluded that he could not easily extricate himself from a commitment and felt emotionally unready to drive alone, with thoughts of impending loss fogging his concentration. I promised that I would ring him later.

That left Ranjit and me.

Whatever happened now, it would be just the two of us.

Having waited for Fr. Erasmus to complete the sacrament and for him to take his leave, the doctor returned to work on Moosh, carrying out checks that I observed in a detached manner and did not comprehend. Once satisfied and certain, he turned to us, introducing himself to Ranjit and then proceeding to explain what we could expect to happen and what would be done for Moosh.

I have, on many occasions, had to impart unwanted news to members of my school community, including sharing news of bereavements. I have seen the struggle for comprehension, the resistance to the truth and the simple, naked devastation caused by my words. I have always sought to handle the situation sensitively and I am told that I have been empathetic, supportive and caring in my manner. That said, I am inordinately grateful that, in my professional capacity, the experience has been rare. I have the deepest respect for those for whom the eventuality is a predictable occurrence and an expected part of their working lives.

In our case, the doctor was the embodiment of practised kindness, as he explained, "Geraldine's vital signs are extremely weak. I am confident in saying, that, should she survive, there will be considerable brain damage.

"I understand that her wish is that no attempt to resuscitate be carried out. It is my view that she is too frail for resuscitation to be safe. I regret to say that Geraldine is exhibiting several of the symptoms of active dying.

"We will do everything in our power to make sure that she is comfortable. I will arrange for her to be moved to a private room, where you will be able to stay with her.

"I know that you have already contacted family, but can I suggest that you update them to allow them to make decisions about whether they can travel to be with Geraldine."

I knew that if Aly had been in the room, she would have asked the doctor to expand on the symptoms of active dying, but my heart was not in it. The element of the doctor's information that transfixed me, had now been stated twice, that there was considerable brain damage.

Thanking the doctor, I turned to Ranjit.

She enveloped me in a forceful embrace, as the doctor left to make arrangements. We moved to sit on opposite sides of Moosh, each holding one of her hands.

"Do you think she is still inside?" I whispered. "Or do you think her soul left, when the Last Rites were given?"

Ranjit shrugged solemnly, stared at Moosh, holding tightly to the hand she had taken, then shrugged again with the faintest smile, "If you're whispering, you must think she can hear you."

"I guess so," I conceded ruefully, before continuing to whisper, "I don't want her to live with brain damage. She would hate that, not that she would know, but she hated the very idea of that happening to her. She found the last few years too undignified, not having full control of her body, needing to be cleaned and tended to. She found the loss of physical capacity and independence difficult enough, not being able to do things she was used to doing, always being expected to ask for help. But this would be too intolerable."

A small part of my own brain vaguely searched around the bed, trying to calculate whether there was something I could switch off to ensure that Moosh was not subjected to living longer, even further incapacitated. I would never have been brave enough to do the deed, but, in any event, I could not fathom out what would work, or, rather, stop Moosh from working.

Ranjit and I were asked to give the staff a short amount of time to move Moosh, so together we went to buy refreshments and for a walk outside. I was sorely in need of fresh air, or at least inner city polluted air, anything that took us away from being cooped up, however briefly.

When we returned, Moosh had been transferred with impressive efficiency to a small room upstairs. Other than a nurse who was present in the corridor, there were no other people in sight or to be heard. There was careful attention to detail in the peacefulness, cleanliness and neatness of the room, with comfortable chairs for us to sit in. And so we sat.

Moosh looked even tinier. She was still alive, breathing, and somewhat disturbing the calm of the room and the equanimity of my mind with her writhing and squirming. Sensing my distress, Ranjit came around to stand behind me, her arms wrapped around my shoulders, her cheek leant against mine from behind.

"She is being looked after very well," she offered. "We can stay for as long as Geraldine needs us."

I nodded, comforted, but not trusting myself to speak.

Suddenly, without warning, Moosh inhaled deeply, a huge, rattling gulp of air. At the same time, she lurched upright in the bed, the sheets falling away. For seconds she was almost vertical, from the buttocks upwards, and then she collapsed backwards onto the bed.

Ranjit and I both leapt forwards. I had my hands on Moosh's shoulders, uncertain what to do, but gently holding her in place.

We looked at each other and I asked, "What just happened?"

"I don't know, but she's breathing. I'm sure of it."

I am certain that Ranjit's look of panicked alarm was a stark reflection of the one on my own face.

"I'll go and tell the nurse and ask what can be done." I said, shaken.

I had no idea what could be done, or whether I wanted anything to be done, but I felt compelled to ask.

Finding the nurse, I haltingly explained what we had just witnessed, to which she replied, "I will come."

Again, I was impressed by the ability to function with calm professionalism and sensitivity in the face of intensely fraught emotions.

The nurse checked Moosh, tidied the sheet over her chest and turned her attention to us, "Geraldine is preparing to take her leave. I like to think of it as taking flight to a place of peace. It is difficult to witness the deep breath that you described, but I must warn you that it may not be the last time it happens. I see that Geraldine has a rosary. You may want to pray with her. I will be close by when you need me."

427

As she left, I must have looked questioning or confused, because Ranjit said, "They will not try to resuscitate, Mark. There will be no more treatment. It is time for us to say, 'Goodbye'. I can't pray, but do you want to?"

I shook my head, holding my arms out to her, silently pleading for a hug.

Inside my head, I was repeatedly telling Moosh that I loved her and that she could, indeed, take flight when she was ready, but I could not express it aloud, not even in front of Ranjit.

Twice more, over what felt like the longest time, but may have been less than an hour, Moosh's body repeated the rigid jerk upright, almost appearing to sit, the harrowing rasp of inhalation driving so deeply into my memory that I can still hear it today. Each time we repeated the nurse's ministrations, neatening the sheet around Moosh and checking whether she was still breathing.

After the third, we waited. We were both breathing deeply, as if trying to inhale for Moosh. I was again repeating inside my head, 'I love you, Ma; You can go now; you are free,' before I realised that Ranjit was holding my arm, her eyes wide.

"Mark, I think she's gone."

This time, Ranjit brought the nurse, who quietly checked Moosh.

For the last time she tidied the sheet and then the rosary beads in Moosh's hands, placing them on top of the fabric. She gently placed her own hand over both of Moosh's and bowed her head. I like to think that she sensed mine and Ranjit's difficulty to pray ourselves and offered her own.

"Please accept my condolences," she smiled kindly. "You are welcome to stay with Geraldine for as long as you would like, or to invite family to join you."

"Thank you ever so much, but there won't be anyone joining us," I said, before adding, "And thank you for being so kind and sensitive with Moosh, Mum. It means a great deal."

She nodded and turned to leave.

Ranjit and I sat, uncertain of what to do, but in my heart, Moosh had already left.

A part of me was delighted for her. No more pain. No more frustration.

A part of me quailed.

With only a nod to one another, we both stood. Ranjit waited next to Moosh, while I went to inform the nurse.

As I turned down the short corridor, a young, Muslim woman was coming towards me, her head covered in a white dupatta. She was followed by two other women, similarly attired. For a moment we both gaped at the strangeness of seeing one another out of context and after several years.

Then, simultaneously she said my name as I exclaimed, "Sabina!"

Both of us realised that we must be on that corridor for the same reason. We were each awaiting impending loss, or the loss had already occurred.

"Geraldine?" she asked, her voice cracking.

I nodded, "Just a few minutes ago."

"May I say, 'Goodbye'?" she asked, uncertainly.

For me, Sabina's presence was the most perfect serendipity. Her warmth had convinced me that Bearwood Nursing Home would be the right place for Moosh. Moosh being looked after by her and her colleagues had given me four and a half more years with Moosh, very often just she and I. Years in which we laughed and cried and grew closer than ever before. Before leaving to become a mother, Sabina had been her ally, the carer who taught her to trust the other carers, the recipient of many Bounty bars.

For Sabina to be present so soon after Moosh's passing, so that it was not only Ranjit and I who were with her, helped me in a way that I would struggle to explain. The human love and tender compassion on her face, as she looked down fondly at her former charge, was beautiful; though I can no longer visualise it, in that moment it lifted me.

Telling the children was ineffably sad.

Poor Alex was separated by distance.

Arun let out an animal howl and ran from the house with his basketball under his arm, needing space.

Ayesha consoled us.

When I rang, Aly was weeping before I spoke.

57

The Tidy Up

Wanting to be as close as possible to Moosh, but now unable to see her at the hospital, Aly came to ours.

Despite our tangentially different experiences of being Moosh's children, we shared our grief.

A part of me was silently stunned that, in the wake of all of the slights, unkindnesses and unfair expectations that she had suffered during her life, as Moosh's daughter, Aly was so broken. Seeing her desolation, but uncertain of when we would be able to see Moosh, Ranjit and I suggested that she stay as long as she needed to.

Seeking to have a concrete focus to anchor Aly, I contacted the nursing home to ask how soon they would need Moosh's room.

They were, as always, lovely, assuring me that there was no rush, to take our time. I took this for the kindness that it clearly was; places there were always in demand. And so, the next day, Aly and I went to the home, very much in a 'Let's-do-what-needs-to-be-done' mindset.

I buzzed the nurse's station and told Sylvia that we had come to sort out our Mum's room. She let us in and we met her at the nurse's station. I have always had a special regard for professionals who do their job efficiently, despite visibly being unable to disguise the emotional toll that their role takes. Looking at Sylvia, it would have been difficult to discern who was more upset, she or us.

She and Aly embraced, sobbing, with Aly managing, "Thank you, Sylvia, for being so kind to Mum, and so caring. You've been wonderful."

"It's been a true pleasure. They don't make many like her," Sylvia smiled through her tears. "She was still doing things her way, right up to the moment she collapsed. Watering her plants one second and then she sneezed and fell."

I am sure that we grinned at that, "That's pretty much exactly how she'd have wanted it!"

"How are you both doing?" Sylvia asked.

"Oh, you know, dealing with things, keeping busy. That's why we're here really." answered Aly, nodding her head towards Moosh's room.

At Sylvia's understanding, sad smile, I added, "While we're sorting through her things, would it be OK if we close Moosh's door?"

When she looked at me quizzically, I clarified, "Mum. *Moosh* is what we called her."

It was Sylvia's turn to grin, "I wish I'd known that. We've never had a Moosh before. Moosh suits Geraldine, somehow. Of course, close the door. No one will interrupt you. Take as long as you need."

Entering quietly, almost reverentially, trying not to disturb

Moosh, I ushered Aly in, clicked the light switch and simultaneously closed the door. Nothing. Or almost nothing. Just a dull gleam.

"It's in nightlight mode. That's going to help! Not!" chuckled Aly.

At first, I could not laugh. I stood in the centre of the room that had been Moosh's home for the best part of the last five years, all 7.5m² of it: a bed, a cupboard, two chairs and a table and an adjoining bathroom containing the toilet (but no escape tunnel). As so many times before, I berated myself that Ranjit and I had not been able to find a way to balance our lives and my career with Moosh's care needs, and that I had allowed a life shaped in an orphanage to come to its end institutionalised, away from her family.

I sank into Moosh's chair. She had loved that chair, preferring it to the much more sensible option of one of the rise and recline chairs that we had tested out. She traced her ownership of it back to being one of a pair purchased by her, one for her and one for Dad, and she had cherished memories of her Siamese, Shona, sitting imperiously on the arm. Not feeling the comforting connection with Moosh that I had hoped for, I found myself rummaging down the sides of the seat cushion, where my hand found several unmistakeable shapes: statin tablets!

"That little minx!" I exclaimed, jumping out of the chair and pulling the cushion out, finally re-finding the ability to laugh. Scattered underneath the cushion, as well as enough statin tablets to have dosed her for over a fortnight, were dozens of carefully snipped *Gods*, and two *E*s. The *E*s were not tablets of drugs but Scrabble tiles. Suspicion caused me to count the tiles in the box, those two *E*s brought the total number in her set to 117 instead of 100.

Aly howled with laughter, "She was always light fingered! Where do you think she managed to rob those extra seventeen tiles from, stuck in a nursing home, never leaving her room?"

"And how could she do this to my carefully calculated Scrabble average?" I wailed. "She's ruined me! It's all been a lie!"

Feeling better for the laughter, I rose to follow Aly's example, joining her in sorting and tidying in the gloom of the nightlight.

In truth, there was pitifully little. I retrieved the array of broken CD players, one for each year in the home: she was always telling me that they did not work, when the truth was that she was, unwittingly, clumsily rough with them. Next, I gathered together the windowsill's worth of the orchids that Moosh had been tending in her last conscious act of life, still stubbornly independent.

Aly pooled items that the home could usefully keep or safely dispose of: boxes of pull-ups, two litter pickers and Moosh's wheelchair and no longer needed pills.

Then she moved onto sorting and folding clothes that I would take to a charity shop, once I felt strong enough to let them go, and it was her turn to exclaim, "Well, what do we have here? That little monster!"

Her eyes were saucers, caught somewhere between genuine laughter and amused fury, as she held her hands out to me. In each she held a brand new bar of Pears soap, still in their boxes, extracted from one of Moosh's safe places that I had not recently visited - they had been tightly wrapped in her pyjamas. All told, Aly unearthed seven bars of Pears in four different 'safe places'. Each new bar made me chuckle and cheered me up, despite Aly's muttered scowls. At each oath from Aly, I offered up a silent apology for all of the times Moosh had insisted that her soap was being stolen.

Aly found not one single Bounty bar.

Years later, thinking back to that day, I would count the two of us inordinately lucky that it was only a stash of *Gods*, Scrabble tiles, pills and Pears that we unearthed, when, on the day of her own mother's funeral, my friend Deb regaled a group of us from school with the tale of searching through her Mum's chest of drawers, in her care home, for the underwear she would be decked in for her final journey.

In the absence of anything even faintly appropriate, to her utter mortification Deb discovered her octogenarian mother's seventeen thongs, all ordered from catalogues. Rather than send her mother Heavenward so scantily clad, Deb gave the funeral directors her own new pair of knickers that she fortuitously had in her handbag.

We were holding back tears of mirth as Deb finished her story saying, " I kissed her on the forehead and told her, 'Look at that, Mum, your bum is as big as mine now!'"

Aly and I each boxed items that had personal connections to our respective families, mainly photographs of the grand-children or gifts that one or other of us had given her, like the cork handbag I bought in Pézenas, which she had kept hanging close at hand but never used. Within my emptied out pull-ups box, now full of frames and bags and goodies that I felt I should take, there was a smaller box of objects that would become my special mementoes of her: a tile from her trip to Jerusalem with the greeting *Shalom*; her collection of crucifixes and a photograph of she and I that my friend, Pam, had framed for her as a Christmas present, the twin of which sat in my office at school.

Last of all, I packed away her box of *God* words with the addition of those found under her cushion and multiple sets of rosary beads in various states of disrepair and El Papa's Prayer Book, still marked at the page she had reached - she had almost finished.

Hugging Sylvia, we ferried the boxes of belongings out to the Zafira. I was crushed, once again, seeing that the meagre collection was not enough to half fill the boot, so, knowing that there was only one potential item that could bulk out our cargo, I told Aly that I would nip back in to make sure that we were leaving the room tidy for the staff to prepare it for the next resident.

Moosh's chair now stood forlornly in her empty room.

Timorously, I stole myself to sit in it again, thinking that maybe we could make space for it in either one of our houses, but it felt wrong. It wasn't merely that, despite all of the efforts to remove the stains caused by spillages and bodily mishaps, the chair was now sorely scarred by Moosh's ownership of it. It was more that, in my head, it symbolised Moosh's imprisonment.

It was the chair that she had been sitting in when I told her that we could no longer have her live with us and that we finally needed to find a home for her, thereby sentencing her back to an institution.

When I was not with her in the home, I always visualised her sitting in the chair, waiting for me, patiently praying.

In many ways the chair highlighted her enfeeblement. She found it difficult to lift herself out of it. Over the years it had more drinks and food spilled down it than I could bare to consider, as she lost control of her hands. Towards the end, it was all that held her up.

Feeling my spirits teetering dangerously, once again, towards a wash of self-recrimination, I told myself that even if I could fit it in the car, I did not want to keep a reminder of Moosh's loss of vitality and autonomy.

In truth, I have frequently regretted that decision, yearning for the solace of Moosh's closeness that I am certain her chair would have afforded me.

Convinced that I could do no more and believing that there was no shred of Moosh remaining, I left, closing the door behind me.

I stopped to thank Sylvia and asked her to pass my boundless gratitude on to the staff, but seeing her emotion flood her eyes, I retreated down the corridor, stopping briefly for a silent, exultant hurrah outside the toilet, in memory of Moosh's most successful escape bid – this was as far as she ever reached under her own steam.

Lastly, I knocked on Mrs. Sandhu's door and asked if she had a minute, wanting to assure her that I would pay Moosh's bill in full, if she could have the final settlement prepared and sent to me.

She welcomed me in.

"Mark, I am so sorry about Geraldine. She was such a special lady."

I willingly accepted what I took to be a genuinely offered platitude, but Mrs. Sandhu continued and her words lifted me from the depths I'd sunk to in Moosh's chair. "Her faith and her determination were remarkable, different, special. I have often told our staff to look at Geraldine as an example of how we must be patient in the face of adversity. I will miss her."

With my heart full, I took my leave and walked to the car balancing my grief that I would no longer visit Moosh there, with my relief that I would no longer see her pain and frustration, and thanking my lucky stars for the night that I turned into that car park to ask if they would be able to care for my mother. They had given her the care that I could not, and given me what they had promised: time to love her, years of time.

I drove Aly back to ours.

I have never returned to the nursing home, despite often wondering whether I would feel Moosh there.

58

The Send Off

Aly was amazing in the run up to the funeral.

She morphed into an organisational she-demon. I did almost nothing, beyond saying, "Yes, that sounds perfect: just as Mum would want it," or simply agreeing to go with Aly's flow.

She arranged everything, starting with the funeral director. As is her way, before I could blink, she was on first name terms with Ann* (* possibly not her real name, as I am useless with names), through whom everything flowed: dates, times, requirements and decisions.

I was summoned, very gently, to a meeting at the funeral home at which we were consulted on cars and caskets, to which I declared that a) I had absolutely no interest; b) I was pretty sure that Moosh would want as little show as possible and c) I was very happy for Aly to make all decisions in that regard.

It wasn't that I did not care; it was that I could not engage, because I could not talk to Moosh about them, now, and we never had done before, that level of detail omitted from our unwritten End of Life Plan conversations. These things just wouldn't have been important to her. Short of knowing, from our plan, that it was of huge importance that we engage a Catholic funeral director, I had no idea.

Fortunately, any gaps in my planning with Moosh seemed to fall into a historic stream of conversation that she had with Aly, down to where to find the documentation for the plot she would share with Dad and what Moosh wanted to be clothed in for eternity. Interestingly, foolishly and tellingly, Aly and I had never merged the details of her conversations with Moosh and my own, until it was too late to seek clarification from her, but I felt able to state, without detriment to my integrity, that I had no knowledge about cars or caskets or funeral tweeds, and did not want to confuse matters.

What we both wanted from Ann* was to know when family members and friends could visit Moosh to pay their respects and say goodbye. In this we were a little ahead of ourselves, as Moosh had not yet been released from hospital, but we were both delighted to hear that there was almost complete flexibility about arranging to visit Moosh, once she was in situ: all that was required was a phone call giving a little notice.

Aly spent some of the time staying with us.

She wanted to remain close to where Moosh was and where she would be brought to.

Our days fell into a pattern of me going to work, Aly organising, and us touching base in the evenings, firstly to go through any arrangements that had been made and then to reminisce.

Some of that was incredibly painful, as our experiences of Moosh were so profoundly and inexplicably different. I was never in doubt that I was precious to Moosh. Even when she sent me away to a junior seminary boarding school, I came to terms with the loss of another set of friends and the chance of finally putting down roots, and accepted that she was doing what she believed was the best that she could for me. Aly has always been more conflicted. At her core, Aly loved Moosh, but there was also a deep well of hurt, resentment and bitterness.

On one of our shared evenings, we were in the garden. It was February and cold, but Aly was having a cigarette, so I had taken my wine out to accompany her beer and we were having a wallow in our loss. In the course of the conversation we recognised that our pain was different. Mine was a simple sense of Moosh no longer being with us: just loss. Aly's was darker, as together we acknowledged that what we had experienced in being the children of our parents had been so markedly different that it had pushed us apart.

I was already shivering before Aly asked, "When this is all done, will we see each other?"

Taken aback, I knew instantly what she feared, "You mean: *ever*?"

Huddled inside an over-sized jumper, her chin quivered, her ciggie hand trembled and her beer hand quaked, as tears streamed down her cheeks. She nodded.

"Bloody hell, Aly, I hope so!" I replied. "Surely that is up to us, now."

"Promise me, Al."

I put my non-wine arm around her to hug her, then

thought better of it and put the glass down to allow a stronger embrace, "I do promise, Aly."

And there it was, the start of a future relationship without either of our parents physically present to complicate things.

Unaccustomed to prolonged shows of affection, I broke away saying, "So, tomorrow night, it's Fr. Guy."

"Yes," she laughed, reassured by my promise and happy to get back to the present.

"You have written your eulogy? Is it four days long?"

My eulogy was a source of annoyed anguish for me.

Ann* had shared with Aly a whole list of *Do*s and *Don't*s for all Catholic Requiem Masses in churches as proudly traditional as the Oratory: things that, most surprisingly, Moosh had been unaware of.

Aly had learned that Moosh's wish for Alex to play Mendelsohn did not meet the stipulation that music at a funeral must be on the approved list of liturgical music. He certainly would not be allowed to play 'Paper Plane', written five years before and so treasured by her - this upset all of us. At least we were reasonably certain that Moosh's choice of hymns would be on the list.

Both Aly and I had been utterly stunned to learn that there was also a strict time limit of three minutes for a eulogy. It seemed that we were lucky to be allowed a eulogy at all, as, ordinarily, it is the priest who delivers a brief homily based on the approved readings and then it is he who gives a eulogy.

This was news that I balked at, vehemently. I had enormous regard for Fr. Guy and the spiritual comfort that his care had provided for Moosh, but I had harrumphed for days about the fact that I wanted our thoughts about Moosh to be expressed by one of us. Even though Aly had secured permission for me to give the eulogy, I was still harrumphing, because there was no way that I could squeeze my thoughts into a measly three minutes.

"I have written it and rewritten it. Would you read it before we go to see Fr. Guy?" I asked.

In truth, it had been mentally compiled and drafted in my brain over all the years since Moosh had first received the Last Rites, and been frequently revisited, revised and, more recently, rehearsed repeatedly.

"I'll read it now, if you like?" Aly offered.

I went up to my office, printed a copy and brought it down, realising that I was assailed by self-consciousness. I was nervous of having tried to capture our feelings. I was also worried that, given our different experiences of her, Aly might not agree with my attempt to extol Moosh's virtues. I put on my coat, collected another can of beer and the wine bottle, as I passed through the kitchen, and headed back to the garden.

I sat and mouthed my words from memory, my breath pluming, as Aly read them for the first time. It seemed to take forever, but I had timed my reading of it at a little short of six minutes. It is possible that intermittent sniffling was reducing Aly's reading speed.

It actually felt as if the joked about four days had passed, when Aly turned glittering eyes towards me from her perch on the step, nodded and said, "Perfect. She'll love it."

I released a sigh of relief, certain that I had been holding my breath as Aly rustled towards the end of her reading.

"Let's hope that Fr. Guy likes it, first," I laughed.

The next evening, I was tense on our drive to the Oratory.

I was not quite girded for battle, as I was far too respectful of the Church to actually seek a confrontation, but I did want to query the barriers to Moosh's non-sacred musical choices and to fight my corner regarding the length of my eulogy and a section of its content.

Even had I been wanting an argument, stepping inside Church House would have quickly quashed that notion. In an understated way the steeped history and sheer size of the building, quietly imposed the power of the Church on the residual vestiges of my Catholocism and brooked no argument.

By contrast, Fr. Guy greeted us warmly, sharing that it was a stroke of luck that he was able to officiate at Moosh's service, as he had only recently returned for a brief stay. He spoke of Geraldine with genuine fondness, before we focussed on the service.

With regret he confirmed that only the hymns that Moosh had listed would be appropriate; no Mendelsohn and certainly not Alex's own composition. I chose to override my rankles that rose at the latter.

We discussed and agreed the readings and the bidding prayers with no issues, before Fr. Guy said, "Aly said on the phone that you would like me to read through your eulogy."

As the minutes ticked by, I once again felt tiny in the large room, my Catholic boarding school days requiring that I accede to the will of the Church. Again, I mouthed my words, willing Fr. Guy to turn the page to indicate that he had at least reached half way.

Eventually, a touch longer than my own best speed, he rested the sheets on the table and chuckled, "That looks like three minutes to me."

Thoroughly grateful for his latitude, but still needing assurance, I pushed "And the last part? Are you OK with me saying that?"

"It is honest and true, Mark. Geraldine will be smiling."

The next few days were a blur.

Ann* finally called Aly to let her know that Moosh had been released to them at the funeral home. We could visit.

After Dad had died almost twenty-five years earlier, I had found it enormously comforting to see him in the hospital viewing room. Moosh and I had visited together. Despite her need of our support, next to his body she had been incredibly strong and loving. I saw that as her visit to Dad.

Ranjit and I had returned a few days later, which was much more for us. I have the most vivid memory of touching Dad's ear lobe, huge and meaty like my own. Although he was cold to the touch, I was comforted to see him at peace and out of pain and by being able to say my 'Goodbye' in private, without onlookers.

Based on that remembered experience, I encouraged the children to visit Moosh, if they chose to. Over numerous visits, items were placed in the coffin with her: twenty years' worth of Palm Sunday crosses; the rosaries that were not being kept as souvenirs; a photo of Dad and a lock of his hair, Ranjit's prayer book gift, and, tucked carefully in one corner, her final God Box including all of the last *God*s from the side of her chair in the nursing home.

Once she had been able to visit Moosh herself, Aly returned to Woodlands and took to directing operations from Loftus, pinging me wordings for Moosh and Dad's joint tombstone, insistent on a reply, despite my assertion that the ground would need to settle, affording us months to decide. Not to be deflected from her mission to have everything sorted, she came back electronically with the draft order of service, asking me to scan specific photos of Moosh that she would include. She double checked that I had contacted everyone on the portion of the list of invitees that had been delegated to me.

I continued to work, asserting that I was needed there. In truth, I would have felt lost without it. Our school being our school, I let the Family of St. James know when the service would be, so that they would be able to hold us in their faith diverse thoughts.

On the night before a Catholic funeral there is the receiving in ritual, when the body of the deceased is brought to the church to lie in readiness. Often this is accompanied by a vigil of the nearest and dearest. Aly had arranged this. The plan was that I would leave school early, pick the family up and drive everyone to the Oratory.

At lunchtime, a need to be with Moosh came over me. I knew that she would be in Church later, but, as I had with Dad, I wanted time alone. Knowing that the HR rule book said that I could have compassionate leave that I had not exhausted and that I could have secured a sicknote and been away from school for weeks, I had no compunction about saying that I was leaving earlier than anticipated. I rang ahead to alert the funeral home. Elaine and Shirley hugged me on my way and promised to join us tomorrow.

I hadn't told anyone else what I was doing: I just wanted to be on my own with Moosh, one last time.

Ann* showed me in saying, "We've kept everything in the

coffin with Geraldine, as Aly arranged it."

As she left me, I turned to Moosh and almost fell over. Sitting in the coffin with her was a stuffed rabbit, all dressed up! If Moosh wasn't there, it would have caused me an unpreventable *What The Absolute Fuck!* moment. I would have to quiz Aly about that later.

My belief system made me certain that Moosh was not within the shell of her body. My lack of faith left me unsure where her spirit would be, and I momentarily wished, jealously, for the religious certainties held by many of my friends. As I had told her, my own take was that Moosh's spirit would remain with me, part of me and part of those whose lives she had touched, Aly, Neil, Ranjit, myself and all of our children. She would be with us in the memories that we held of her. I believed that knowing her and being moulded by her would influence us in our future lives.

So, as I sat with her, I gathered my own memories of her to me, to be treasured. I touched her gnarly hand that had so often reassured me and then I bowed to kiss her on the forehead, lovingly and protectively, for one last time, thanking her for all of the love and blessings that she had bestowed on all of us.

When I left her, just as I had been at so many important moments in my life, I was buoyed by that love, knowing with certitude that I would continue to carry it with me.

Upon arriving in the Oratory car park, just short of 4 o'clock, to await the hearse, I was stunned to see that many staff from school had raced from work, or taken time on their day or afternoon off, to come to pay their respects, joining other friends, who knew that they would not be able to take time

447

off work the following day.

When I expressed my surprised to some of the women from school, they answered, "Where else would we be?"

Their unexpected presence and their hugs meant the world to me.

Only flashes of the funeral service come back to me.

I remember that I was calm, efficient, controlled and a little detached. I remember greeting parishioners from the Oratory, who I recognised, before we made our way into Church. I remember Aly standing to walk to the altar for her reading, accompanied by Jess. Touchingly, she had asked Jess to be next to her, while she read, to give her strength and comfort. I remember Dominic forfeiting the chance to pre-read our chosen text, by arriving late, due to traffic, but striding forward and delivering the unseen reading with such perfect gravitas that I could hear all of our deceased school masters offering celestial applause. I remember approaching the pulpit with confidence, in the knowledge that Fr. Guy had sanctioned my eulogy, and speaking lovingly about the strength that Moosh's faith had given her, particularly in the years of her illness.

And I remember looking across to Fr. Guy before ending by saying, "Those of you who know me well, know that my belief system is different from Mum's, but I find myself able to say that I have faith that she is where she wants to be and where she prayed she would be."

I was pleased that the cemetery was fuller than when we buried Dad. I sent a quiet apology to him for the fact that this was only the fourth or fifth time that I had been back since his funeral. I knew with a great degree of certainty that I would be an even less frequent visitor in the future, as two of my visits had been to bring Moosh. I am profoundly respectful in graveyards and am appalled when I witness other people not being, but, for me, they are not where I choose to remember my loved ones, or to pay my respects.

We laid Moosh to rest exactly where she had planned to be, with Dad.

After the prayers were said and the last of the graveside hugs and condolences were gratefully received and everyone had made for the cars, I stood next to what was now *their* grave, my mind going back to my conversation with John, almost five years earlier.

Deep inside, I was gratified. I knew that I had done everything that I possibly could do to help Moosh. I hated Parkinson's, the illness that had robbed her of so much, but I knew that, strangely, it had given us time, she and I.

Since the disease had brought her to live back in Smethwick, first with us and then, for much longer, in the home, there had been so much laughter and so much joy. In amongst her frustration and discomfort and the challenges of attending to her needs, we had bonded more closely than at any point in my life. In the hours that she and I had shared, particularly once the home's abundant care gave us such freedom, there had been so much fun, so many more moments with her grandchildren than we had dared hope for, those unexpected pleasures of seeing Sandra and Kay again, and, for the two of us, so much closeness and so much love.

And so much Scrabble, because to one little, old lady, approaching the end of her life, Scrabble = Love.

Moosh and I had been, in the strangest of ways, truly blessed.

59

The Bar Tab

I had grown up believing that funerals are disconsolate, onerous occasions and, of course, they *are* imbued with feelings of loss, regret and devastation. However, as I have become older and, as happens, attended my share of funerals, I have come to the conclusion that they have the potential to be joyful and uplifting.

Some are truly remarkable occasions.

After the formalities of Moosh's Requiem Mass and burial, I was gratified that we had fulfilled almost all of Moosh's wishes. From funeral home, to choice of Church, to Fr. Guy acting as celebrant, to being reunited with Dad, Aly and I had followed Moosh's instructions. But, it could still have been lonely and unremarkable.

Moosh had lived an itinerant life through over half of her marriage and had set up our family home in those fourteen different houses by the time Dad died. From their travelling years, she had kept in touch with just three friends, two in Canada and one in the UK. Moosh never experienced family life until Aly and I came along, having been separated from her parents as a two or three-year old and placed in the convent orphanage. She had lost touch with her older sister for over half of their lives and her younger for long periods. Sandra was far away in Malaysia and unable to join us. Although reunited for a fortnight in their seventies, on Moosh's great adventure of reconnection, Marguerite was not well enough to travel from Adelaide, and would soon pass away herself, hopefully to enjoy a raucous reunion and everlasting sisterly mischief, beyond the Pearly Gates. Pamela, her single remaining, devoted friend from her convent days was in Singapore.

Having first been institutionalised in the convent and then being reclaimed by extended family to perform questionable duties of servitude, Moosh had lived almost the full first half her life being unwanted. She was used to relying almost entirely on herself. After Dad passed away, Moosh had not been a hermit exactly, but she was very content to live a private, insular life on her road, enlivened by her visits to mine and Aly's homes to be with the grandchildren whom she adored.

Up to her final years being cared for in the nursing home, Moosh's main point of social contact, beyond us, had been Church and a number of her parishioner friends had stayed in contact, asking for news and occasionally visiting her, although they were beset themselves by life challenges of their own.

As a result, there were precisely zero family members beyond Aly and I and our immediate families at the funeral, no friends pre-dating Moosh's move to Shakespeare Road and only the smattering of parishioners that we were still in contact with. It should have been one of those sad, depressing passings, a quiet shuffling off with almost no fanfare . . . it turned out to be anything but.

Despite the small, not wanting to say tiny, pool of candidates who might be able to join us, we decided to hold a wake for Moosh.

We had known that we would be joined by our local friends and dear friends from my school days, Moosh's friends from Church, and Shirley and Elaine from school. We knew that Ayesha's friend, Hannah (aka Quad) would be coming to support her. We knew that several friends would be travelling a distance to support us and to remember Moosh. We thought it only proper to provide food and an opportunity to catch up and thank them.

Unsure how many would appear, but not wanting to underestimate, we booked The Kingshead, who would put on a finger buffet for us and make sure that they had enough of Ranjit's favourite wine at a reasonable price. Ranjit and I were a little conscious that the bulk of people who had said they could come were on our side, but Aly generously assured us that the more the merrier and suggested pulling people in off the streets to bulk up the numbers. As it turned out, that would not be necessary.

While I had been standing reflecting next to Moosh's grave, Ranjit and the children had waited at the Zafira. We had urged those who had come to the cemetery with us to go ahead to the pub, as well as suggesting to those who had to return to work that they join us later in the day. We also knew that there were other friends who were not able to take time off from work for the funeral but wanted to come later to support us and to pay their respects, which we were looking forward to.

By the time we arrived, the formal shroud of the funeral rites was already dispersing. Dominic greeted me by engulfing me in a hearty hug to check that I was coping, and I applauded the admirable gravitas with which he had delivered his reading. He was followed by a procession of others, who also wanted to be sure that we were not overwhelmed by the sadness of bidding farewell to Moosh.

Once it was clear to all that we were bearing up, the room relaxed into knots of conversation and mini reunions of those who had not seen each other recently, in some cases decades. And, with that, began the most joyful and entirely unexpected afternoon of storytelling. One after another, as we rotated around the room or they came to us, friends shared their tales of Moosh.

Brian and Dominic had memories going back to the 70s of her coming to school. She could never come on the official Visiting Sunday, so would turn up whenever she was in the country to take a group of us out for a meal, Dominic relishing the wickedness that he was able to get away with when the rest of us would be scolded.

Never to be outdone, the grandchildren got in on the act, led by Liam and Alex going through what seemed like hours of tales of making Moosh laugh, either at their inappropriateness and daftness, or of them laughing at hers. They told the stories of the non-moving orange fish, re-enacted their entire David Attenborough routine and howled about the time that Moosh had adamantly and repeatedly claimed that there was a black man sitting in the corner of the room with her and Liam's friends, only to be told that it was in fact a guitar case leaning against the wall. The stories kept coming, until I and others pleaded with them to stop to allow us catch a breath.

Arun, Ayesha and Quad added stories of their own, of pizzas and sandwiches being hidden behind the kitchen radiator and of visits to see her at the nursing home. Moosh's projectile dentures featured in several of their yarns, but it was Ayesha's relating of her last time with Moosh that captured the mood: with Moosh having difficulty speaking, she and Ayesha were ribbing each other in actions and facial gestures. Seeing Moosh's tongue protruding from between her dentures, Ayesha mimicked her. Not to be outdone, Moosh apparently thrust out her tongue a truly horrifying distance, causing them both great hilarity and giving Ayesha a memory to tuck away against future need.

Teresa (a good Catholic girl), Sally (an Anglican reader) and Shirley (a Sikh) all shared recollections of visiting Moosh in her weaker years, speaking of the faith that they had witnessed and the emotional strength that had moved, impressed and inspired them. I had always been deeply grateful when friends with faith visited Moosh, opening windows of conversation that I felt were closed to me, and affording Moosh the succour of shared or parallel spirituality.

Finding myself briefly with Aly, we hugged and congratulated each other on how well things were going and then, fortified by a couple of glasses of merlot, I asked her about that rabbit.

"Oh, that's Harvey!" she announced airily, as if that made it crystal clear. Seeing my bemused expression, she went on, "Like the film. Jimmy Stewart. *Harvey The Rabbit.*"

I know I must still have looked perplexed, as Aly finally gave in, "I made the bunny for Moosh. She loved it. It was bigger than expected, so Moosh named it Harvey, not after Harv, but after Harvey the six foot rabbit in the James Stewart film. She loved that film too. She said she'd always keep Harvey and said that he should go with her."

The two glasses of merlot must have worked their magic, because that all made perfect sense to me.

Throughout the afternoon, well-wishers came and went, each one lifting us, either with stories of Moosh or, much more simply, through their compassion and love. After many of the longer distance travellers had headed off on different motorways, the workday ended, which heralded a further wave of hugs and kindness and friendship. We felt truly blessed.

First came colleagues from mine and Ranjit's schools, keen to pay their respects. Heading back down the stairs from a comfort break, I became aware of Aly in the centre of a throng of my friends from school, who had surrounded her *en masse* and declared her to be an honorary member of The Family of Saint James. Aly falls instantly in love, but never more so than that afternoon, when it became obvious to her that Moosh's progress had been followed so closely by this group of people, who had never met our mother, but, out of concern for me, had cared about her.

Shortly afterwards, I became aware of a sizeable group that we had not factored into our plans (or my budget). Arun, who had possibly struggled the most in the immediate aftermath of Moosh's passing, had sent out a text message to his closest friends letting them know that I intended to buy a drink for every person who joined us and urging them to come. Cue Team Azza, a collective of ethnically diverse brotherhood. We had seen them grow from boys to young men, taken them to countless football matches and had them around at our house for adolescent shenanigans. We had been there in the fallout of countless boyhood and early manhood scrapes, but now Arun had need of them and here they were to support their friend, with admirable maturity, the free beer an entirely unnecessary incentive. To their absolute credit, each of them came to find Ranjit and me to offer their condolences, to give me a manly handshake and Ranjit a huge hug.

The bar tab came to £871, for which I blame Arun entirely.

As we, somewhat hazily, wended our way home, congratulating ourselves on a) choosing a venue within walking distance and b) the utter genius of dropping our cars at home earlier, we all reflected that Moosh would have been delighted to have been so well remembered.

For a funny little soul, who kept herself to herself, she had touched many lives and engendered fondness in more people than we had imagined.

60

Afterwards

Initially, I didn't cope especially well, once the day of Moosh's funeral and wake had passed.

For me, the final physical loss of Moosh, was simply the culmination of all of the steps of loss that had begun with her stumbles on the school run with Ayesha. We had been losing her, incrementally, for a long time and witnessed her struggling with her loss of herself.

I was convinced that she was in a better place, not in terms of the spirituality that I spoke of in church, but that it was better for her to no longer be suffering. She had hated it. So, I was at ease with that.

I was fine with the functional, administrative processes such as tidying up finances, acting as joint executor to the will; sorting out probate; ensuring that bequests were made. All of those aspects, despite being new to me, were similar to the decision making and procedure following that are part of my working life at school.

My difficulty rested in my inability or refusal to grieve.

School became my focus and my excuse for not mourning. I took just one day off work on the day after Mum died and another for the funeral. Beyond that, I took no more time, arguing that school needed me (and probably convincing myself that it would tumble without me). It was true that we were fighting hard to reach the standards expected of us and it was true that meeting those challenges was taking a great deal of creative and strategic energy, but I allowed myself to become much more obsessively school-fixated than ever before. As each wave of grief rolled over me, I consciously crushed it, telling myself that my job required that I stay focussed.

One evening, months later, Yeeshy, who was about to turn seventeen, sat next to Ranjit to confirm that I was being irritable, short tempered and sometimes unreasonable. Kindly, she reassured me that I wasn't being scary, but that she, they, felt that they were losing me and had no idea how to reach me.

What I would not tell her then, because I felt that she was too young, and what I would not tell until I acknowledged her as an adult, is that the suicidal urges had returned and that I was fighting hard to hold on. At the forefront of my brain, school was dominating and overwhelming me and the fact that headteacher friends were losing their jobs for not reaching the dreaded standards was causing me to feel increasingly exposed and vulnerable, professionally. Much deeper inside, I was no longer crushing the grief, it was smothering me. I yearned for Saturdays at the nursing home; struggles with dentures; random herbal remedies; *Murder She Wrote* and Scrabble. I missed having my biggest fan willing me on and reassuring me, the woman who had always told me that I could be or do anything I wanted. Conversely, I was avoiding driving down the Bearwood Road, so as not to pass the window which was no longer hers.

I was dangerously adrift and losing all sense of having an anchor to hold me here.

On the day that Yeeshy spoke to me, it was three weeks since my most recent suicide urge, the one that I had most fully prepared for, down to date, time, location, method, organisation of the things I'd need and who would find me. Thankfully, so thorough was I in my preparations that, at the point of setting pen to paper to draft the five notes that I would leave, I terrified myself and confessed to Ranjit. I gave into her pleas to seek professional counselling. It was almost certainly the best money that I have ever spent.

Seeing the counsellor enabled me to release my emotion, my loss of Moosh and my sense of embattled powerlessness at school. The initial outpouring in her room was, for me, an embarrassing catharsis of wretchedness, tears and snot. But it allowed me to rationalise the pressures and challenges at work and to be less anxious about the implications of our school's vulnerability to poor data. I only visited the counsellor once, but that one session saved my life: the suicidal drive receded and it has never returned.

Crucially, the counsellor helped me to create emotional space to reengage with Moosh, to hear her advice and to apply it. It was she who used to counsel me, "Don't bottle things up, Alistair. You try to carry the weight of the world, and all of us, on your shoulders. You don't need to and it's not good for you. Let it out."

And so I do.

Rather than crush emotion and pain, I have learned that what works for me is to allow myself time to release it. When I become aware of the build-up of the longing or loss, rather than barricading it behind an internal dam, I intentionally pierce the barrier, usually by watching a film or listening to music. I have never been much of one for anniversaries. I don't miss Moosh or my father at Christmas or on their birthdays, not even the first one after each of them died, and I rarely register the anniversary of either of their passings. I am, however, prone to those moments that have become Facebook clichés, when you just need a Mum Hug. They do not happen so often now, but in moments like those, when the longing is strong, my go to film is *Field Of Dreams* – it has never failed to dissolve me to relieving tears. There are songs that have the same effect; I'm soppy like that.

We are each of us different and so we approach life in different ways, including bereavement. Consequently, I know that my approach of accepting the pain and riding its wave would not be for everyone, but when friends lose those precious to them, my advice to them is to celebrate their loved one and to cry: to actively remember, to carefully catalogue and cherish all of their happy memories and, if (when) they need to, to cry like a drain.

The only other very clear piece of advice that I find myself offering to those who find themselves in a similar situation to Moosh's and mine is: use the time to capture their threads. We were so fortunate. We knew that there was a risk that Moosh would reach a point when she did not recognise me or lose her capacity to communicate. We made sure that we talked. Often it was utter nonsense, but at other times we talked deeply and I delved into her memory banks of family. Still, if I had the time again, I would be much more systematic about devoting more of our time to asking even more questions about her family history, to fill my gaps.

I loved Moosh more and loved her better from the moment of Aly's phone call on the night of Ranjit's birthday party than at any other point in our lives. Faced by the many challenges and sadnesses catalysed by her disease, together the two of us had found a way to gather precious threads, some vivid and richly evident to be gleefully grasped, others gossamer fine, but no less rich, to be carefully captured and tenderly harboured: the multiple kindnesses shown to us; the loving support of friends, family, professionals and the wonderful staff at the home; Moosh's indomitable spirit and her deep well of faith; and our ability to find fun and laughter in amongst the distress and pain and trials that Moosh faced.

Between us, sometimes intentionally, but also by good fortune, we had woven those threads into a peculiar but life enhancing kind of joy.

It might be strange for a son to write a love letter to his Mum, but, fortified by the joy that we wove in those five years, this has been mine.

VII

Part Seven

Eulogy
March 2012

61

A Tribute To Geraldine (My Eulogy)

While writing *Who Stole Grandma?* I searched for the eulogy that I had written for Moosh's funeral. Despite having had laptops that died and USB sticks that became corrupted, I found it in an email to Aly, to whom I had given the paper copy, as I left the pulpit in the Oratory, and who had lost it before reaching home.

Tribute to Geraldine

To most of you Mum was Geraldine or maybe Mrs. Lanyon, when she was being posh. To Ayesha, Harvey, Arun, Liam and Alex she was Grandma. To Alyson, Ranjit, Neil and myself she was Moosh. Last week I found out, for the first time, how to say her birth name, Sudanamee, a lovely Hindu name.

Mum was born a Hindu, baptised an Anglican and then, at the age of three, given into the care of a Catholic convent in Malaysia. Three belief systems by the age of three!

Initially, Mum became a Catholic by default, when she was abandoned into the orphanage that was part of the convent. She and her sister, Marguerite, were accepted on the understanding that they would be brought up as Catholics. For mum, this was a life-defining event in so many ways.

Out of the desolation and hurt of being placed in the orphanage, and through the care of the nuns, Mum grew to embrace the Catholic faith. Throughout her life, Mum's Catholicism was of central importance to her. It guided her and comforted her through a life that was so often touched by hardship, loss and mistreatment. Whatever life threw at her, she met it with the faith that God would care for her.

As a mum, she had the ability to believe ludicrously positive things about us. For most of my teens mum was particularly taken with the notion of me being an Olympic gymnast! Do I look like an Olympic gymnast? She supported Alyson and I time and time again, bailing us out and taking great joy from our successes.

As so many parents do, Mum came into her own as a grandparent. She was devoted to her grandchildren, and absolutely loved that last 22 years, celebrating their different strengths and successes. Alex acknowledges that, without her inspiration, he would never have developed the musicality that is so central to his life. Liam always had the power to make her laugh with his easygoing personality. She loved reading newspaper reports about Arun's football matches and she loved meeting Ayesha's friends, like Quad, who would visit her. She was especially besotted with Harvey and simply showered him with love. It also gave her enormous joy that Liam had found such happiness with Jess and I'm certain that she will be present in spirit at their wedding.

As you know, Mum's last decade was blighted by Parkinson's Disease. I hate Parkinson's Disease with a passion. Mum hated it too, because of the loss of physical capacity and, towards the end, the difficulty in communicating fluently but, as so often before, her faith sustained her. She devoted much of her time to prayer, dismantling any number of sets of rosary beads! She used her faith to argue against the well-intentioned risk assessments that the staff at Bearwood Nursing Home put in place in their attempts to stop her from falling and putting herself in further danger. She would patiently explain to them that to not use her legs to walk, when God had given her the strength to, would be wrong. Mrs. Sandhu, the manager, told me that she used to tell her staff to look at mum as an example of how to be patient in the face of adversity. She certainly tested their patience! But they were brilliant and so was Mum! She was still defiantly pulling doors off cupboards to the end and her last conscious act was caring for her plants.

Mum kept showing us her love right to the last. She recently re-found the ability to write, which had eluded her for much of the last few years. In her last fortnight she painstakingly wrote a lovely and loving letter to Alyson to console her about Neil's mum's illness.

Despite her loss of capability, Mum retained her sense of humour. On her last Wednesday, the day of Ayesha's last visit, Mum was too weak to speak properly, but she and Ayesha were teasing each other through actions. As she was leaving, Ayesha spotted that Mum's tongue was sticking out a little and teased her again, to which Mum stuck her tongue out a truly disgusting amount, causing them both to giggle a lot. I'm so grateful to her for giving Ayesha that last memory.

Ranjit and Mum had an interesting relationship from the starting point of Ranjit failing the Irish Catholic test and Mum being a classic demanding Indian mother-in-law at heart. In her weak moments, however, Mum admitted to loving Ranjit and being very grateful for her support. It's possibly true that Mum's love for her was at its height on her last full day of life, when I gave her the Pope John Paul II Prayer Book that Ranjit had *bought for her from the Vatican. She was glowing and she very nearly finished reading it.*

For seven years I was under strict instructions from Mum to ensure that she received the Sacrament Of The Sick, if she was close to dying. I do not know what the world record is but Mum received the Sacrament five times. I am so pleased that there was time for Fr. Erasmus to come to City Hospital to give Mum the Sacrament one last time and for including us in the ceremony. As Fr. Guy says, she was "Good To Go". Those of you who know me well, know that my belief system is different from mum's, but I find myself able to say that I have faith that she is where she wants to be and where she prayed she would be.

On behalf of Geraldine's family, I thank you all for holding her in your thoughts and prayers.

When I found my eulogy, I had already written several of the chapters that are referenced in it (Grandchildren and Other Visitors; The Risk Assessment(s); El Papa's Prayer Book) and so, when I read it again after an interval of over six years, I was delighted that my memories married with my tribute to her.

Acknowledgements

Over the two and a bit years that it has taken me to draft *Who Stole Grandma?* (and then tinker and procrastinate), I have owed thanks to several people.

Firstly to Aly for going through the pain barrier with me: I regret that her pain was far, far greater than mine. Our memories of certain events vary almost as widely as our experiences of being Moosh's children, but she has read and reread *Who Stole Grandma?*, offering corrections and different recollections, but, most important of all, giving her blessing for me to share this story. I am enormously grateful to her.

And to Aly and Nelly, together, for giving me time to start my writing at *Casa Abajo De La Cueso*, looking out across a stunning valley filled with serried ranks of silver-grey olive trees, basking in November sunshine: it was exactly the time and space that I needed.

To Charlotte & Nick for their emergency hospitality, and to Charlotte for sharing her experience as a memoir author. Writing chapters overlooking Iznájar was a special treat, particularly when it twinkled at night.

To Jen, Bob and Jayne for allowing me to invite myself to their beautiful piece of Languedocian paradise, to finish writing chapters of *WSG?*, just as I had started, looking up from my keyboard to stare across a stunning vista. I have been incredibly lucky.

To all of Team Moosh, (Aly's Family and mine) for sharing their reminiscences with me and allowing me to adapt their words to my own. In some ways, the writing of *WSG?* made hers the longest wake ever, but it was lovely to have you as part of my thinking.

To Auntie Sandra, for our text messages back and forth to make sure that I was clear on the content of Chapter 45: the story of she, Ball and Balraj tracking down Moosh.

To Sandra, Kim and Teresa for being the first non-family readers of *Who Stole Grandma?*, for their validation and suggestions, and to the followers of my Facebook blog *The Adventures Of The Reluctant Retiree*, who were my audience in my first venture into self-publishing, for all of their messages of support, for their gentle prods and suggested corrections, for sharing how *WSG?* resonated with them and, crucially, for their encouragement to share this story more widely.

To Debbie, John and Foxou, for giving me their gate code and their internet password and an open invitation to make myself comfortable and post instalments every day for 24 days straight.

To Dari at Reedsy Editor for helping me, a mildly stressed technophobe, to navigate a completely new (to me) writing tool and answering my entry level questions, as if I was a proper writer.

To the 33 friends, some of whom I have never met, who put their hands up when I needed help with the final proofread. I was staggered by their generosity of time and grateful for all of the checking that that they instigated. Any mistakes that remain are mine alone.

To Ameesha at The Book Shelf Ltd. for taking on a publishing novice and offering kindness, critique, advice, guidance and encouragement, and hand holding me through the process of getting *WSG?* to you.

Crucially, to Her Most Wonderfulness, Ranjit, for her patience in finding things to fill her hours, while we were at our Little Tin Shed, near the sea, so that I did not feel guilty writing, and then again back at home, when the rewrite took much longer than expected. Her quiet reassurances of, "I'm enjoying myself, you do your work," allowed me to finish drafting . . . and redrafting. Her pride in the first sharing of *Who Stole Grandma?* and her emotional investment in its telling touched me deeply.

Like Aly, HMW is central to this story: she suffered unfair treatment from Moosh, but, like Aly, she said, "Bring her here."

Most of all, I thank her for the love she showered on me, when she knew that I was struggling in my darkest twelve months. I'm not struggling anymore.

Lastly, I have no idea why I gave Ann* an asterisk to acknowledge that Ann was not her name. There are several people beyond our family, who appear in *WSG?,* whose names I changed, either because I forgot their given name, or had not asked their permission to include them. Any character given a name, either their own or one I created, benefitted Moosh's life in some important way, so if you find yourself reading this and think, 'That's me!', *Thank You* from Moosh and from me.

May 2021

About the Author

Mark Lanyon enjoyed an itinerant early life, as his father's soldiering took his family around Europe and the UK, before attending a junior seminary boarding school in Staffordshire, then teacher training college in Birmingham.

Now an ex-teacher and head teacher, he is relishing a much needed retirement, a part of which was always going to be devoted to writing this story and several more.

When he isn't writing, Mark can usually be found being a besotted Grandad, or exploring country walks in the UK, or cycling through vineyards in France, always taking photographs, *or* embroiled in shenanigans with his wife, Ranjit, and their retirement buddies.

If you would like to find out more about Mark's writing, please visit https://marklanyonstoryteller.com

Printed in Great Britain
by Amazon

62698057R00286